HELP ME! I'M LOSING MY SIGHT!

CRITICAL TIPS AND TECHNIQUES TO HELP YOU COPE WITH VISION LOSS

DARLENE G. SMITH

Published by Nonie's Korner
P.O. Box 2442
Freeport TX 77541
www.NoniesKorner.com

Smith, Darlene G.
Help Me! I Am Losing My Sight!
Critical Tips And Techniques To Help You Cope With Vision Loss

ISBN: 978-0-578-17137-1 (paperback)
ISBN: 978-0-578-17138-8 (ebook)
LCCN: 2016909795

Interior design and production by J. L. Saloff, www.saloff.com.
Front cover by Mark Saloff Designs.
v.1.01

Disclaimer:

The information contained in this book is for informational purposes only. Any advice given is based on the author's personal opinion and experience. You should always seek the advice of a professional before acting on something that has been published or recommended.

The author and publisher shall have neither liability nor responsibility to any person or entity with respect to any loss or damages arising from the information contained in this book. Every effort has been made to provide reliable information and links, which are subject to change without notice, and which is beyond the control of the author.

ACKNOWLEDGMENTS:

I would like to give all my thanks to my Lord and Savior Jesus Christ for helping me every step of the way and his continued support and blessings.

Contents

Introduction

If you are in the first stages of losing your eyesight, or you have a progressive eye disease that is robbing you of your vision, access to practical knowledge is the key that will enable you to successfully manage your day-to-day activities with confidence and ease.

Please allow me to introduce myself to you. My name is Darlene and I have been dealing with diminishing eye sight for over forty years. I was diagnosed with the juvenile form of macular degeneration when I was just 12 years old. I am now much older, and have learned many ways to cope with my dwindling vision.

When you have an incurable eye disease and have been to the ophthalmologist as many times as I have, it is not a very pleasant experience. At my last appointment I was diagnosed with the initial stages of glaucoma and a little cataract thrown on top for good measure. I felt very frustrated with the diagnosis my doctor had given me. If you do not know, macular degeneration destroys your central vision and glaucoma claims the rest.

As I was contemplating feeling sorry for myself, the nurse assisting me in the examination room told me about her mother losing her sight due to diabetes. She told me that her mother was having a hard time adjusting to her vision loss. This is not the first time that I was told of someone losing their sight who did not know how to deal with their prognosis. Most people are at an older stage of life when diagnosed with an eye disease, which makes it even more difficult to know what to do or find what resources are available.

Since I have had a lifetime of experience successfully coping with my own visual challenges, I had considered writing an informative guide to help others struggling with theirs. My conversation with the nurse was the final push I needed to move forward with this book in order to help the vast number of people facing eye conditions that are likely to cause them significant vision loss. Over the years, I have developed and learned an abundance of tips and tricks from my own personal experience coping with macular degeneration. I can clean my home, make a wonderful meal for friends or family, get to the grocery store, and shop, all with little or no help.

In this book we will discuss many topics, such as our home and how to take care of it. I know that transportation is a concern, so we will look at different ways to get around. Together, we will review medical tools and techniques that will keep you safe and healthy. I will share the gadgets, gizmos, and simple strategies that have helped me stay independent and virtually free from frustration throughout my life. I am confident the information that I have provided will ease your fears, so you can successfully manage all of your daily challenges.

For example, there is a vast array of tips and techniques that you can use to find things and complete tasks as they arise. In one instance, a friend of mine was riffling around in her hand bag trying to locate a bottle of nail polish. As her temper started to blossom, I told her to feel for the shape of the bottle without actually looking. She found it immediately and was truly amazed that she could use her touch and not her eyes to find it so easily. Now she uses this simple technique when trying to find things in her bag even though she has perfect vision.

I understand the overwhelming feelings of devastation and uncertainty when facing a visual disability. My personal turning point came when I accepted my condition and put my faith in my Lord God who has given me the strength and courage to be the best person that I can possibly be. You can choose how you feel each and every day. You can get up and be in a negative frame of mind or you can have a positive one. I choose to be as positive as I possibly can.

Regardless of your sight, you can succeed! You can do anything you set your mind to. Do not let an unexpected curve in your life send you barreling over a cliff. Coping with vision loss will be frustrating at first, but with a little help from this book, and the love and support of your friends and family, you will feel great about yourself and things will get easier.

So on that note, come with me and let us take a journey together through the pages of this book. Relax, take a deep breath, and let us begin.

1

Mobility and You

❧

Personal mobility and transportation are two of the most important issues we face in our daily lives. Just like other people, we need to go to the grocery store, the doctor's office, the dentist, and many other places. It is very frustrating when you are unable to drive yourself where you need or desire to go. We still want to retain our independence and successfully arrive at our destination by ourselves. There are several ways to accomplish this goal. Let us take a tour of the different types of tools and services that are available.

Mobility

I want you to know from personal experience that the very best mobility tool is a white cane made specifically for the visually-challenged. This cane will help orientate you to your surroundings and allow you to walk with a great sense of safety and self-assurance. When using the cane properly it will warn you of obstacles in your path and keep you from tripping over them. It will help you manage curbs and stairs, particularly when maneuvering down them.

Using this cane will boost your confidence and allow you to be more independent. I know that your friends and family will also enjoy your company to a greater extent, because they will not worry about you as much when you are walking around by yourself with the help of your cane.

The Americans with Disabilities Act protects visually handi-capped citizens from discrimination. In addition, it specifically gives the right-of-way to any person carrying a white cane. Using the cane will alert other people that you have difficulty seeing and assure that they move out of your path. Generally, they will be more helpful and aware of you especially on side-walks near busy streets.

If you need a cane, the National Federation for the Blind (NFB) can provide one free of charge. You can contact the NFB at 410-659-9314 to start the process and fill out the required forms.

If you have a cane but do not know how to use it, you can con-tact the Division for the Blind and Physically Handicapped in your area and they will help you. Usually the Blind Services will send an experienced mobility instructor to your address and you will receive one-on-one training on how to use your cane to assist with mobility and orientation. I guarantee that you will be walking with a great sense of confidence when you are using your cane because you will not be afraid of tripping or falling in unfamiliar territory. If you qualify, the Division for the Blind will provide this and many other blind-associated services to you free-of-charge.

Did you know there is a day set aside for people using the white cane? On October 6, 1964, Congress designated October 15 of each year as White Cane Safety Day. This day celebrates the con-tributions and accomplishments that blind Americans achieve every year and the independence a white cane can provide.

Some people are embarrassed to use any type of mobility device, especially a cane. They feel as though it detracts from their appearance or draws attention to their limitations. This is just plain silly. If a cane or other device will help you get to your destination safely, use it! I have had friends fall and hurt them-selves and even I have taken a few spills in my life. I am too old for that now and will use anything to help me get around safely and so should you!

Another amazing mobility tool is a guide dog. Under the Amer-icans with Disabilities Act, a guide dog may accompany you any place that you want or need to go. The trainers who work with these animals from the puppy stage up until a blind person receives one should be commended for all their hard work and dedication.

Before I tell you about receiving one of these dogs, I want you to understand that these animals are not pets. You must be able to dedicate time and energy to it and be responsible for maintaining his or her training. You have to be able to feed and care for your dog. This includes being able to walk with it for exercise and bathroom breaks, and especially being able to keep up with its veterinary visits.

Please do not let me discourage you from getting a guide dog if you truly need one and can devote the time and resources necessary to keep it healthy and trained. The service and companionship these animals provide are truly extraordinary.

There are twelve schools accredited by the International Federation of Guide Dog Schools in the United States and many more in other countries. To receive a dog from one of these schools, you must first meet the qualifications for their program. After you have met this requirement, you must complete the proper paperwork and wait for approval.

Once approved, you must attend the school for the crucial one-on-one training, which lasts about one month. Upon arrival, the school will assign you a guide dog and teach you how to care for it. Instructors will help you become acquainted with your new companion and teach you how to let your dog guide you safely and independently. Your companion will help you maneuver around obstacles, navigate stairs and curbs, and can even help find different objects. You and your new friend will work together and learn many things.

The dogs know how to manage elevators and bus stops as well as how to help you locate the entrance to your home or a building. They can even assist you in finding your mailbox and so much more. Just remember that while the dog is guiding you, you are the one in charge.

The cost for training just one animal can be over $25,000 but the cost to you is virtually free. Unfortunately, the government does not fund the cost of training guide dogs and these programs depend on grants and loving donations. Please let your friends and family know about the great need for donations to support these awesome schools.

Check with the Division for Blind and Physically Handicapped for more information or you can also search the Internet to find the school best suited to your needs.

Transportation

Driving a car is one of the hardest things to give up when your eyesight starts to fail because of the overwhelming sense of freedom and convenience it provides. Unfortunately, you will reach a point when your limited sight makes it unsafe for you to drive. When you get to that point, please stop. If you continue to drive after your eyesight makes this activity unsafe, you will put yourself and others in grave danger.

I heard a story concerning a man who continued driving even though he knew he should not. One day, he drove through a school zone and stopped because a little boy was trying to cross the street. The man in the car waited patiently for the boy to cross the road but all he did was stand there. The man grew impatient, got out of the car, and called for the boy to hurry across the road. When the boy still did not move, the man approached him and found to his utter dismay that what he thought was a boy was in fact a fire hydrant. Embarrassed and glad no one was there to witness his mistake, the man drove home with great care and never got behind the wheel of a car again.

This is just one example of people still driving after it has been time for them to quit.

Although you will no longer be able to drive, you do have many other options. The Americans with Disabilities Act gives people with disabilities many important rights in the area of transportation. If you are disabled, you are entitled to the same right to use and enjoy any type of public transportation as people who are not.

For example, one very important source of transportation is the public buses available in and around large cities. When onboard a bus, the driver should assist you if you need any help. They are required to announce every stop audibly so if you have a problem understanding what they have said, ask them to repeat it. Do not falter, because helping you is part of their job. In addition, you should be able to get your bus passes at a discounted rate. Call the office of the specific bus line that provides transportation in your city for more information.

Under the Americans with Disabilities Act, if the local transit authority cannot adequately serve you through its regular bus system, it is required to create a parallel transportation service. This service specifically meets the needs of individuals with disabilities who are unable to get to and from the local bus due to their handicap. Eligibility for this program is based on the existence of a functional limitation that prevents the patron from walking or rolling to a bus stop.

When using this parallel transportation service, you should be able to schedule a trip and be picked up at your door, taken to your destination, and returned to your home. You should be able to schedule a ride twenty-four hours in advance and your pick-up time should be within one hour before or after the time you requested. Call your local city bus system and they will be able to help you with eligibility and any further details you require.

If you live in a city that has subways, trains, or any other type of public transportation I have not listed, be sure to contact your local transit authority and they should be able to help you with whatever information you need.

In some cities, accessible transportation may still be a problem but there are places you can get in touch with and ask for assistance such as the following:

- The Lions Club assists people with visual limitations. Your local chapter should have volunteers that will drive for you if you make the proper request.

- The Red Cross will provide rides for your medical needs if you have documentation showing you have a handicap from your doctor or another reputable source.

- The Department of Health and Human Services might be able to help you with information concerning van pick up in your area and any other transportation options available in your community.

If you have a smart phone, you can download and access several app-based car services such as Uber, Lyft, or Gett that might be found in your area. These ride-based services are similar to taxies and I would strongly suggest you research them. You can find consumer reviews with positive or negative trip time, cost, driver courtesy, and other important tips to make an informed choice.

When addressing transportation needs, do not forget your friends and family. Every one of them has to venture to the grocery store so why not accompany them? Do not feel as though you are a burden because they would most likely enjoy your company. Just ask in advance and I am sure you will have all of the rides you need.

Another alternative to finding transportation is to advertise in the newspaper. I chose this option while I attended a college in Houston and lost my steady driver. The university is about 60 miles from my home and I desperately needed a new ride. Incredibly, one of my neighbors answered my first ad. This was a wonderful turn of events because we were not acquainted at the time but have since become the best of friends. I attended school for over three years and found five drivers by advertising. This taught me that where there is a will there is a way.

Help Me! I Am Losing My Sight!

You do not know what you are capable of accomplishing unless you try! Do not be afraid to reach out of your comfort zone. You have resources available to you, but you are the one who must be diligent and find them.

From time to time, you might have to travel by an airplane to get to your destination. When arriving at the airport, go to the curbside porter and check-in booth for your particular airline. It is typically located by the entrance doors of the airline on the "Departures" level. Give the porter your identification and flight information and ask for assistance. An airport employee will guide you through the security line and take you to your gate. If you need a drink or snack, just ask and they will be glad to assist you in buying it. When arriving at your gate, the employee will make sure the airline staff knows that you need help boarding the plane. Upon arrival at your destination, the flight attendants will help you deplane and find someone to assist from there.

One tip: if someone is picking you up at the airport, ask him or her to meet you at baggage claim. This makes it easier for the airport employee who is helping you find your party without any hassles.

Airports can be very big and confusing so ask for assistance from the airport staff to help you get to where you need to go. They are familiar with the facility and can help you find your way. When all of these issues are addressed it will improve your frame of mind and make for a more relaxing and enjoyable trip.

Before I end this chapter, I wanted to share a funny story about myself. One night my friends invited me to accompany them to a local bar and grill. After a few hours in this establishment, I was ready to go home. I said my goodbyes and went outside to call a taxi.

When I called the service, the dispatcher told me it would be about ten minutes before a cab would arrive. I waited outside for fifteen minutes then called the taxi company again. The dispatcher promised me that my ride would be there any time. I waited another ten minutes and called a third time. This time growing impatient, I asked again, where is my taxi? The dispatcher assured me that the car was just pulling into the parking area. She asked me to stand where the driver could see me and that he would pull up right next to me. I promptly stepped to a place that I felt sure he would easily see me and I began to retrieve the money for the cab. While I was trying to find my money, a car with writing on the door pulled right beside me with his back door right in front of me. Of course, I opened the door and got in.

I looked up in utter shock and amazement to find that I had climbed right into the back of a police car. I could not believe it! The police officer was just as amazed as I was. He had never had anyone willingly get into the back of his car while on duty. I told him that I thought that his car was a taxi. He promptly informed me that this was the easiest arrest he had ever made. I told him I had made a big mistake. I showed him my money for the cab and told him that I was visually impaired. He let me out of the car and both of us had a good laugh. I thanked him and bid him a safe night.

At that exact moment my friends who I had accompanied to the establishment came out the door. When they saw me outside they told me to get myself over there and they would take me home. On the way home I explained to them what had happened to me and they had a big laugh too. This has become one of those blind stories that always entertains and amuses everyone.

So the moral of this story is do not stay cooped up in your house because you are blind or losing your sight. Staying home can make you feel depressed and lonely. So get busy and find the transportation you need. Go somewhere fun and enjoy yourself! You might end up experiencing an incredible moment, as the one I did, and have a great story to share that will have everyone laughing, too!

2

Magnification and You

❧

In this chapter, I will discuss a variety of low vision magnification aids that I know you will find exceedingly helpful in managing your day-to-day activities. When you first realize that you are losing your eyesight, it is crucial that you try to maintain and enhance the vision you still possess. I think that you will be delighted with the assortment of products that are available to help us accomplish this objective.

 The first thing I would suggest is that you obtain an appointment with a good ophthalmologist who specializes in low vision assessments. Your personalized assessment will determine which low vision aids best suit your condition and activity requirements. Since low vision optical devices are task-specific, the doctor may prescribe several different types of visual aids for your vision needs.

Help Me! I Am Losing My Sight!

There are specific devices for:

- Reading a book or newspaper

- Viewing your favorite program on TV

- Spotting bus numbers or street signs

- Watching a football game, concert, or a play

If you do not have the income to afford these devices contact the Division for Blind Services in your area. They may be able to help you obtain a low-vision evaluation to determine which magnification aids that will enhance your vision.

You can use magnifiers to increase the size of fine print in books, magazines, newspapers, and any other small print. There are handheld magnifiers that range from 2x to 22x in strength. This means that the object you are viewing will be enlarged by the amount of "x" times your magnification device has. For example: 10x strength equals the object being enlarged ten times.

If you need to use both hands to work on a project or hobby, there are larger magnifiers that incorporate a stand. Handheld and stand-mounted magnifiers can also be purchased with a built-in light which can help your vision immensely. Also, if your hands are unsteady the stand version is a good choice because you do not have to hold the lighted magnifier in place.

One thing I have learned is that a higher strength of magnification may not be the best solution. For example, I love to play poker with my friends and we use the jumbo print cards which you can purchase in any discount store. I have a 7x lighted, hand-held magnifier that I use when I play. I thought if I used the 11x I would be able to see much better, but that was not the case. There is a smaller field of view with a higher strength of magnification, and the higher strength did not work for me at this time. So my advice to you is to schedule an appointment, visit a low vision center, and check out all of the different strengths of magnification aids that are available. Magnifiers come in all shapes, sizes, and strengths so you can pick out the ones that work the best for you.

If you have specific things you need to see, take them with you to your low vision evaluation. This will help you determine the aids that best suit your current eyesight. One important point I would like to make is to please take your time when choosing your new vision helpers. Do not let anyone rush your decision. These aids can be relatively expensive and you might select more than one. If you are not sure about a specific device or magnification level, wait and think carefully about what is going to work the best with your sight. It might be a little overwhelming if you have to choose more than one item at the same time.

Remember, different vendors may have different products and the prices and usability might vary from one product to another, so be a smart consumer and check out all of your options.

Another type of magnification product is a magnifier that will enlarge your computer monitor or television set. These are large magnifiers that are mounted on a stand that you place right in front of your screen. If you are just starting to lose your vision, this might be a great alternative to purchasing a larger TV or monitor. For example, the magnification can turn a 32 inch LCD flat-screen TV into a 38 inch, saving you money. These magnifiers are great because they are inexpensive and very easy to set up. An Internet search will identify several sites that carry these great magnifiers.

A monocular or a pair of Binoculars can be a great tool for see-ing objects in the distance. The monocular is made for one eye and the binocular has lenses for both. You can purchase these in different magnification strengths according to your need. If you have macular degeneration or another chronic eye disease that causes a blockage point in your vision, a monocular is the best choice as you do not want one eye competing with the other. Try each of these and see which one best enhances your sight. Both of these options can be great tools and can be very light weight and manageable. If you have children or grand-children, this will be a great investment for you as you can keep a watchful eye on them from a distance.

If your hands are unsteady, a handheld binocular or monocular may be difficult to use. In this situation you have an option of having the lenses mounted in a pair of glasses. I have been introduced to people with low vision who are still driving safely by using this type of mounted monocular. Consult your eye doctor for more information about this very important subject.

One of my favorite visual aids that I use every single day is a closed circuit television (CCTV), also called an electronic video magnifier. This device is extremely helpful for people gradually losing their sight because it can be adjusted as their needs change. This visual aid consists of a video camera that displays a magnified image on the built-in CCTV viewing display, computer monitor, or your TV. There are five basic types of video magnifiers: desktop models, flex-arm camera versions, head-mounted display designs, hand-held camera to TV types, and a variety of portable and pocket models.

The CCTV can magnify a word from 1x up to 100x depending on the capabilities of the screen you are using. You can purchase them with a color display so your pictures will be in true color. They can also provide a good color-contrast in black or white. I like reading on a black background with white letters, because it is easier for me to see. I can read my mail, look at a magazine, or reminisce over old photos whether they are in black and white or color.

The handheld option is a good choice if you need to use it away from home because it is small and very manageable. Some of them have a camera that flips up on the side so you are able to sign your name on a line with no trouble or guess work. There is also a freeze frame option that allows you to pick up the unit and take a closer look at what you are viewing.

If you are interested in one of these units, many of the vendors will bring their products directly to your home where you might be more comfortable. An in-home presentation will allow for a one-on-one experience so you can determine which of the versions work best for your needs.

For better price options, check with the doctors, low vision clinics, and vision rehabilitation agencies that may offer a loaner program or resell pre-owned machines in your area. Also, check on e-bay or any other websites, such as Blind Bargains, that might have pre-owned merchandise which could substantially reduce the purchase price.

Another product that you should try is a selection of colored acetate sheets which you can purchase at any office supply store. Colored acetate sheets can be an inexpensive alternative to other devices if your eyesight is still relatively good. When placed on a page, these translucent sheets, especially light blue, yellow, or marigold, can enhance the contrast between the print and background, making words and letters appear darker and easier to see. You can also cut them to fit the book or magazine you are currently reading, and they make a great book marker.

If you enjoy using a computer, there is a magnification program already preloaded in its system. The Disability Discrimination Acts of the US, UK, and Australia require that all computers have accessibility software programs in their systems which can be accessed from the control panel. If you are not computer-savvy, get someone who is familiar with them to help set it up. Also, additional magnification programs will be discussed in Chapter 3.

Technology is constantly growing, evolving, and transforming our lives for the better. Cutting-edge products are being developed every day, so do not miss something extraordinary. For example, today I was watching my local news and learned about a new magnification aid that just might change my life and yours. Developed by eSight, these electronic glasses allow people who are legally blind to see most things that normally -sighted people see such as:

- People's faces, from up close and afar

- Newspapers, books, menus, signs, and other reading material

Help Me! I Am Losing My Sight!

- Computers and other work-related tools

- TV, movies, and other entertainment devices

- Concerts, plays, and other live events

The eSight glasses are completely mobile, which means users can experience all kinds of activities such as:

- Going for walks

- Participating in sports

- Working with computers and other work-related tools

- Reading signs and other navigational markers

- Watching outdoor events

- Using public transportation, including air travel

eSight glasses will enable us to enjoy so many activities we are not able to do now, maybe even driving. Before you consider these glasses, you must have some remnant of vision that eSight can electronically enhance.

One obstacle is the fact that these digital electronic glasses are not cheap, but there is help available through their website or you might be able to find funding yourself. Check out eSight at www.esighteyewear.com or call them at 1-855-837-4448.

This is why I am so adamant about you staying informed and educated. You have to be your own best advocate in anything you do and information is definitely the key.

I hope this chapter has answered most of your questions about magnification and its immense benefits. Just remember that patience will be needed when you receive your new low vision devices. It takes time and practice to master the use of any unfamiliar piece of equipment. Insist on being properly trained in the use of each of your new vision aids until you feel comfortable with their operation. Low vision rehabilitation is an ongoing process, so if you find that the device you were given is no longer helping, you should schedule a new low vision evaluation with your doctor.

3

The World of Technology and You

Technology has exploded on to the scene with a vast selection of innovative products that have made a huge difference in everyone's lives, but is extremely valuable to the visually-challenged population. With these technologies we can grow in knowledge, reach great heights of independence, and open new doors filled with hope and opportunity. We are truly blessed to be living at this time in our history. Do not be afraid to venture into the new world of technology because your life will become enriched in ways you can't now imagine and you will not want to live another day without it.

Computers and Other Amazing Technologies

The most indispensable form of technology that can help us every single day is a computer. Computers enable the visually-challenged to virtually leave their homes without depending on any type of transportation. You can travel to a store and do your shopping. You can travel to your bank or post office. You can chat with people from around the world. You can even find a date online or form an online business by using a computer. If you have a question that needs an answer, the computer can quickly find the information you are seeking. You can even further your education online. There is an abundance of great things you might be missing if you are not taking the time to learn and operate this amazing tool.

You might think you are not able to use a computer because of your eyesight, but this is simply not true. There are magnification software programs available that will enhance the size of the images and words on your screen up to 36x (36 times). This is a very large image at full zoom. The magnification program is designed to work like a magnifying glass as it moves over the page you are reading. If you have a chronic eye disease that is diminishing your eyesight gradually, this is a wonderful software tool as it will adjust to your vision as your eyesight declines. You can zoom in on any image for a larger and better view.

You can also manipulate the contrast and colors on your computer monitor to best suit your visual needs. ZoomText (from Ai Squared) and MAGIC (from Freedom Scientific) are two of the most popular screen magnification software programs available.

Help Me! I Am Losing My Sight!

If your eyesight has progressed to the point that you cannot use a magnification program, there are speech programs that will enable your computer to speak everything that appears on your screen. The software can be set to English or any other language you want or need. Its purpose is to make computers accessible to blind and visually-challenged users by providing you with access to the information displayed on the screen.

The program reads everything aloud making it possible for us to independently use the computer whether it is at home, school, college, or our workplace. It allows for comprehensive keyboard interaction so you do not have to use a mouse. JAWS for Windows created by Freedom Scientific, Window Eyes developed by GW Micro, and Super Nova designed by Dolphin are just a few screen readers you should check out. These have similar software programs so you will need to research them and figure out which one you are most comfortable using.

Each of these screen readers is unique in the way it operates. The key strokes you use to do a certain task can be completely different from one software program to another. You can download a free sample demo of these products by going directly to its vendor's website. This is a great idea, because you can get the feel of each of them.

When choosing your new software, you need to take your time and explore all of your options. Remember: if you purchase a magnification and a speech program separately, make sure that they are compatible and can run simultaneously. The magnification software can also be purchased with a speech-ready application. This is why you must be the one to determine which program you like the best: magnification-only, speech-only, or magnification and speech.

Another type of software program is called scan-to-speech. This program can turn written text into synthesized speech. Scan-to-speech uses a scanner and software to scan printed material and read it aloud. You can scan your mail, your bills, a cookbook if you need to read a quick recipe, a newspaper, or most any text, including money. There are portable units that you can take with you where ever you need to turn written words into speech.

This is a great tool if you are going to school because it will scan your text books, a test you need to take, or anything you have to read. Using this program you can do the work right in the classroom without feeling left out or unable to do the assignment with the rest of your classmates. In the work environment, this is truly a Godsend as you can read any necessary documents to complete your work accurately and independently.

The two main scan-to-speech software programs are Open Book by Freedom Scientific and Kurzweil 1000 by Kurzweil Educational Systems.

Help Me! I Am Losing My Sight!

Back in the day before these technologies were available, I attended a local community college to further my education. I was taking a few classes including a business course. The very first session of this course, the professor asked the class to go to the library. She wanted us to read a magazine article and write a thesis on what we had read. Knowing I would be unable to do the work in the library, I ask her if I could take the magazine home. I explained to her that I was visually impaired and needed a personal reader to read the article out loud to me so I could accomplish the task. Without any type of understanding, she calmly told me, "If you cannot do the work when I ask, get out of my class." Feeling very inadequate and embarrassed, I did.

This just shows that throughout your life time, you will encounter people of this ignorance. Do not let someone like this keep you from fulfilling your dreams. In today's world of technology, you will be able to do anything you want or need to do as well as any sighted person. Equip yourself with the right technology and the education you need to operate it correctly, and there will be no stopping you!

For more help and information on these wonderful software programs, contact the Division for Blind Services in your area. You can also contact the vendor directly if you have any questions concerning their particular product. The Division for Blind Services can help train you to successfully operate your computer. They can provide you with the means to learn the current Windows applications and the important speech and magnification programs that will help you operate your computer as well as any sighted person.

You do not have to feel trapped at your home when you have a computer that you can operate successfully. You can travel to where ever your imagination can take you. All you have to do is learn the computer, equip it with the proper software programs, and get onboard the World Wide Web.

Cell Phones and Apps

Cell phones are another amazing form of technology that have been a monumental source of help in our lives as the visually-challenged. They have enabled us to have a greater sense of independence because we have the capability of using a phone at any time we need. But one of the most important uses for a cell phone is being able to call 911 in case of an emergency situation. Section 255 of the Telecommunications Act requires that phones must be available that are readily useable for people with disabilities.

There are currently two manufacturers of magnification software programs for your cell phone: Code Factory and Nuance. These magnification programs can magnify the text on your cell

31

phone screen up to sixteen times (16x). You can also manipulate the colors on your screen to create a better visual contrast. Just remember, the higher the magnification the less text will be visible on the screen.

If you need more than a magnification program, there are currently three manufacturers of screen reading software for cell phones: Code Factory, Nuance, and Dolphin. These software programs work like a computer screen reader such as JAWS or Window Eyes when installed on your cell phone. You need to make sure your phone has a compatible operating system and that the magnification and/or speech software works with your phone. The manufacturers have this information available on their websites or you can call them directly. These software programs give you full access to all the features and functions that are available on your phone.

With technology advancing so rapidly, a computer-based smart phone has become one of our best options. A smart phone might be a little more complicated to operate, but after you get the hang of it, I think you will love it for all of its great features. This type of phone is virtually a small computer with its speech/magnification capabilities accessible right out of the box.

The main way to interact with these phones is through a variety of specific gestures made with your fingers on its touch screen. After consulting with my blind friends and exploring all of my options, I decided to purchase the iPhone. I was told the iPhone included an innovative screen reader and other accessibility features that made it easier for the visually-challenged to operate.

I was a little intimidated at first because I was not familiar with any of the touch screen commands. I got on my trusty computer, did a search, and found a very informative instructional book to help me get comfortable using my new phone. The book is "Getting Started with the iPhone: An Introduction for Blind Users," written by Anna Dresner and Dean Martineau and it is published in print, Braille, and DAISY text by the National Braille Press. This book will help you understand all of the features and functions available on the iPhone so you can successfully start using it. The phone number for the National Braille Press is 1-800-548-7323. In addition, check with your cell provider about their free classes that will teach you how to operate whatever smart phone you choose. And finally, do a search on the Internet to find an assortment of good information to assist you.

A smart phone has the capability of accessing the Internet and making it possible for you to download a number of blind-friendly apps. Apps are applications created specifically for computer-based phones which can provide them with additional useful functions that can help you every single day. For example, with these apps you can search the web, blog, contribute to your twitter and Facebook account, or play an exciting game.

There are apps that can:

- Teach you various subjects or help you with school assignments.

- Record your heart rate over a period of time and then send this information directly to your doctor.

- Track blood sugar levels, which can be useful if you are diabetic.

- Determine the color of something.

- Scan a bar code on a product and immediately tell you what it is.

- Read your money.

- Read a menu, newspaper, or other text.

- Help you find your way home if you are lost.

These are just a few examples of apps available that can make your phone into a very rewarding and powerful tool. Make sure you stay knowledgeable about the brand new ones being developed that will benefit your life and independence.

To find any blind-friendly app, go to the app store on your phone and do a search for "apps for the blind." A number of apps will appear for you to consider. Make sure you read the reviews, especially if you are paying money for it. Some of them are great and function as they are intended but others simply do not work.

Other Technologies

One of the products I really love is a talking caller I.D. Plug the unit into your home phone and when it rings you will hear the number of the person or company who is calling. You can also personalize your caller I.D. with the names of your friends and family and it will then say their name when the phone rings so you will know immediately who is calling. A lot of the new land-line phones have this function already built into them and are available through many of the big box stores.

Another fantastic product that has revolutionized our daily lives is a talking bar code reader. Virtually everything you purchase today has a bar code. Wouldn't it be awesome if we had a technology that would recognize the bar code and read it to us out loud? Well now we do with the I.D. Mate Galaxy created by

Help Me! I Am Losing My Sight!

En-Vision America. This scanner can be used to quickly identify any product or item that is not easily recognized, such as jars, cans, boxes, bottles, clothing, playing cards, prescription drugs, books, CDs, DVDs and so much more.

Many of the products contained in the data base have extended package details, such as ingredients, warnings, instructions, package size, nutritional values, song titles, movie ratings, and miscellaneous package details. This scanner is lightweight and portable which makes it very easy to take anywhere. The UPC database updates are available every six months so you will be able to add more products to its data base.

If a product does not have a bar code, additional bar code labels are available for purchase. Adhesive, tag, and clothing labels can be placed on nearly anything you need to identify. After attaching the bar code, you can record a short description of the item and know exactly what it is the next time you pick it up.

There is also a new, smaller voice labeling system called a PenFriend. It is in the shape of a pen and is created by RNIB. It allows you to record information onto self-adhesive labels that you can then place on any dry goods, foods kept in the refrigerator or freezer, all paper work, and you can even keep a diary. There is no limit to the record length associated with each label which makes it easy to have a detailed description of any item you need.

You can find these and other similar readers by doing a search on the Internet. Also, contact the Division for Blind Services in your area to obtain a one-on-one demonstration.

If you have problems determining the color of things, a talking color detector is a great item to add to your arsenal of helpful products. Color identifiers are portable devices that enable people who are blind, visually impaired, or have a color vision impairment distinguish the color of cloth, paper, plastic, or other natural products. They announce all the common colors, plus many tints and shades.

Color Teller by Brytech and Cobalt Color Detector are two of the many devices on the market. Some of these units have an assortment of functions such as a light detector, clock, calendar, thermometer, voice recorder, and much more. So, no more excuses for mismatched socks!

Another extremely important form of technology you should be using is a currency reader. The Franklin Bill and the Orbit iBill are just two of the numerous handheld portable talking money identifiers available. These readers enable the visually challenged to immediately determine the amount of money they have, ranging from a one dollar bill to a one hundred dollar bill.

Help Me! I Am Losing My Sight!

This is essential, because you will not have to ask someone else for help identifying what bill you have in your hand or if you are receiving the correct change when making a purchase.

It is very sad, but the U.S. Treasury Department has never designed or issued paper currency that people with poor vision could easily recognize until The American Council of the Blind filed a lawsuit. The suit claimed that the Treasury Department violated the Rehabilitation Act of 1973, which was enacted to ensure that people with disabilities can live independently and fully participate in society. As a result of the ACB's legal victory, the US Bureau of Engraving and Printing (BEP) will now provide FREE currency readers to persons with vision loss. Contact the National Library Service for the Blind and Physically Handicapped (NLS) or call 1-800-424-8567 and they can assist you.

If you are not a patron of NLS, you must fill out an application and have it signed by a competent authority, i.e. your ophthalmologist, who can certify your visual impairment and then submit the form to: www.bep.gov/uscurrencyreaderpgm.html. In 2020, there will be other changes to the U.S. currency to make it even more accessible to us.

I believe this is one of the most valuable chapters in this book because these technologies are so critical to our independence and sense of wellbeing. You must unequivocally try to acquire all of the products and skills it will take to help you thrive in your daily environment. Do not tell me you can't because you are too old, you do not have the intelligence, or you do not have the money. It might not be easy, but anything worth having is worth the extra effort you put forth to obtain it.

4

Your Health and You

❦

Your health is the most important thing in your life. Regardless of whether you can see or not, if you do not have your health, you do not have anything. If you find yourself thinking that you are no longer able to manage your own medical needs, relax because there is an assortment of products and systems that will enable you to accomplish this goal.

The one thing that I would like to stress to you is to please try not to worry about every little thing. Life sends us many obstacles to test our faith and endurance. You must stay strong and try not to brood over every challenge life throws at you. This stress alone can cause you a myriad of different health problems. So take a deep breath, try not to worry, and let us venture forth to see what is available to help us stay healthy.

Managing Medications

If you are like me, you're taking some kind of medication, whether it is a vitamin, an aspirin, or a doctor's prescription. If we're taking more than one type of pill, it is crucial that we know which one we are putting in our mouths. We do not want to make a mistake and take the wrong one. There are many ways to create an effective identification system for our medications, so let's review the various options.

If you are taking only a few medications, the most effective way to identify them is by the shape of the pills, such as round, oblong, or rectangle. Capsules and tablets are also easy to distinguish from each other by their texture and feel. You must practice feeling the different pills in your hand until you can easily recognize them. Ask your pharmacist about the different shaped pills that you might be able to get in the same prescription you are taking. I was able to get a capsule instead of a tablet in the same exact medicine I was prescribed. This made it easier for me to determine which pill I was putting in my mouth, because I was not taking any other medications in capsule form at that time.

If you are taking different medicines during the night and day, separate them by putting the nighttime medication in or on your bedside table and your daytime ones where you hang out during the day. Store your bottles in zip lock bags to protect them and keep them together. You can separate your night-

41

time and daytime medicine into two different bags. Make sure that wherever you place it, the pills are not accessible to children or pets.

When opening your medication, place it over a container with raised sides, such as a tray or a cookie sheet. This will keep you from losing any pill that you might accidentally drop.

If you are taking medication on a daily basis, you might be able to identify your medicine by the shape and size of the bottle they are in. One bottle could be bigger than another, or the bottle could have a distinguishable shape that makes it easy to recognize. There are also many ways to mark your bottles so you can identify which medications they are, including:

- **Rubber Bands.** You can place different sizes or thicknesses of rubber bands around the bottles for easy identification. Use one size rubber band for the first bottle or two thicker bands for the second. You can mix them up by putting one thin and one thick on it or two thick and one thin. Use the system that works for you.

- **Tactile Dots.** Place a tactile dot on the lid or on the side of your prescription bottle to help identify it. Bottles can be labeled in braille or large print using Dymo or label-on tape.

You can also use glue or a 3-D Pen. Just write the first letter of the medication name on the lid, and after it has dried, you can easily read the raised markings with your fingertips.

- **Duct Tape.** Stick a piece of duct tape on the bottle and mark the first letter or the first few letters of the prescription with a thick, black felt pen for identification. Be sure that you do not cover the medication label. Select duct tape in a good contrast color such as white to make it easier to see the black writing.

Remember to save your marked lid or bottle and put it with your new prescription. This will keep you from having to mark a new one every time you get your prescription filled.

- **Magnifiers.** Use a low-vision, lighted magnifier if you are still able to read your labels this way.

- **Large Print Labels.** Ask your pharmacist to use large-print labels on your prescriptions. These are available at many pharmacies but most visually impaired individuals do not know about them because they are not readily advertised.

In addition to the options above, there are also several types of Talking Prescription Readers you can use. This device allows you or a pharmacist to record up to a minute of detailed instructions and precautions on its digital recording chip. These reusable readers attach to the bottom of most standard sized pill bottles. After you receive your reader, take it to your pharmacist and explain how to record your prescription information on it. I am sure he or she will be happy to do this for you. While there are various vendors for this product, one choice is manufactured by the Millennium Compliance Corporation and is available through the National Federation for the Blind (NFB). Contact the NFB at 410-659-9314 for more information.

Some of the major chain pharmacies such as Walmart, Rite-aid, and CVS have made talking medication labels available for free through their stores and En-Vision America. En-Vision America created the script-talk station so you would be able to read your prescriptions comfortably at home. Simply press a button and place the special Talking Label over the reader and all of the printed information will be read aloud. Because the data is stored in the label itself, it can be used on any size bottle, box, vial, tube, or other prescription container. For more information on how these labels work and to have your pharmacy participate in the Scrip-Talk program, call En-Vision America at 1-800-890-1180.

Another way of storing your medication is in a weekly or monthly pill dispenser. This allows you to separate your pills into daily doses, even if you are taking your medication more than one time a day. This will also enable you to know if you have taken your medicine, and if so, how many doses. In addition, you can purchase some pill organizers with a dosage alarm which will remind you when to take your pills each and every day. Likewise, some medication organizers can be obtained with large print labels in a contrasting color. The labels can have writing with black on a white background or white on a black background. You can choose whichever contrast works the best for you and your visual needs.

When dealing with liquids and creams, do not forget your other senses! You can usually identify these products by their texture or smell. You can use the same methods shown above to identify these containers as well.

When picking up your prescriptions from the pharmacy, make sure you are getting the right medication. It is important to have someone check your prescription labels at the time you pick up your medicine. First, ask them to read the label aloud so you can be sure that the prescription was correctly filled. Second, open your medicine and check the pills. If they do not feel like the right ones, ask your pharmacist about this. It is very important to ask rather than to take the chance of taking the wrong medicine and ending up in the hospital or worse.

For example, I heard a story about a man that was prescribed an eye drop. He used it for several days with each drop causing him more pain. He later learned that he was given the wrong medication. He was putting ear drops in his eyes, and actually lost his sight in one eye due to a pharmacy mishap. So, be smart and check your medicine!

This next product is the I.D. Mate bar code reader. This is a wonderful tool to help you read your medication whether it is prescription or over the counter. It will literally read the bar code to you, telling you exactly what you are holding in your hand. If your medicine does not have a bar code label that is recognized by the I.D. Mate, you can create one and attach it directly onto your medication bottle. Then just scan the label and record the pertinent information into the bar code reader's memory. The next time you scan that medication it will recognize it and tell you which medication it is, as well as the recommended dose, precautions, and any other applicable information you have recorded.

I absolutely love this product and raved about it in the Technology chapter of this book. I know that a lot of you may not be able to afford an I.D. Mate, but look for refurbished ones and like-new bargains on the low-vision websites. I knew of someone buying one on eBay for virtually pennies on the dollar. He was very lucky and maybe you will be, too.

Managing Diabetes

An increasingly common disease found in today's world is diabetes. This prognosis can be emotionally devastating for someone with vision loss. Not only are you facing a diagnosis of a chronic illness, you are also dealing with adjusting your lifestyle and daily habits to manage it. Do not be afraid because there is help available to you.

Visually-challenged diabetics can continue to be independent and confidently take care of their own diabetic needs. The blind can and do accurately draw up insulin, monitor blood glucose levels, and complete other diabetic management skills just as well as any sighted person.

If you are dealing with diabetes, The National Federation of the Blind (NFB) will be a great help to you and a good source for diabetic information. The NFB established the NFB Diabetes Action Network (NFB DAN) which improves lives through advocacy, education, research, technology development, and programs encouraging independence and self-confidence. If you want to be part of a caring support group that has a great source of information about diabetes, the Diabetes Action Network is a great network for all diabetics, especially those who are blind or losing vision.

The NFB Action Network also publishes a magazine that focuses on nonvisual methods of managing this disease. It is called the

"Voice of The Diabetic." Each issue contains personal, candid stories written by diabetics, friends, health care professionals, and others who share their experiences and expertise on diabetes and its complications. This magazine emphasizes the importance of good diabetes control, proper diet, and independence. The features of this magazine include a medical Q and A column, a "Recipe Corner," and a resource column of aids and appliances. You can listen to this magazine over the telephone through the NFB-NEWSLINE for free. You can find the NFB at: https://nfb.org, or contact the NFB-NEWS LINE staff at 1-866-504-7300. Also, go online and check out all of the services offered by the NFB for diabetes self-management and a whole host of other important topics dealing with blindness.

Blood Pressure and More

If your doctor has asked you to keep an eye on your blood pressure, there are monitors that will read your diastolic and systolic pressure out loud, and will also give you a reading on your heart beats-per-minute. This can be a very useful tool if you are suffering from hypertension. Most of these machines will keep a record of your daily readings and you can easily take it to your doctor's visit where he or she can review your pertinent information.

A talking temperature thermometer is a very important device to have on hand in your first-aid kit. It will enable you to monitor any fevers that might pop up in your family so you can act accordingly.

Manage Your Weight/Health

The best strategy to stay fit is to maintain a healthy weight. If you are needing to lose a few pounds, there are many recipe books available in audio, large print, or in a braille format. You can also go online and find all kinds of recipes and weight-loss support that will help you achieve your goal. There are talking kitchen scales for portion control, as well as talking weight scales that can help you track your progress. A talking pedometer is a great tool to help keep track of every step you take in a day. Exercise is the most important thing you can do for yourself. Not only will it help in your weight loss goals, it will also help you get in shape and stay healthier.

Do not let your eyesight keep you from joining a gym or an exercise class. Many gyms have personal fitness trainers and often include a free introductory session with one of them when you join. These trainers will establish an exercise program that is designed to help you achieve your fitness goals. All you have to do is be brave and ask for help.

The machines might be a little intimidating at first, but once you get familiar with them, you will be exercising like a pro. The exercise equipment is placed in a certain format in every gym. The machines are quite heavy, so they should be in the same spot every time you go. This makes it easier to get orientated and familiar with the gym and where each of the machines are located. Every piece of equipment has the raised location dots so you will be able to easily adjust and use each of them. If the raised location markers are not to your satisfaction, bring your own tactile dots and put them on the machines you like to use.

I know you can exercise at home, but going to a gym will give you more of an incentive and you will meet new friends with the same goals in mind.

If you are dealing with a chronic eye disease that is disrupting your vision, you should really consider taking vitamins that are made specifically to promote good eye health. Your daily eye-defense multi-vitamin regimen should contain vitamins A and C, lutein, Zeaxanthin, and zinc. Also, make sure you eat a lot of green leafy veggies because they contain a great source of vitamins and antioxidants which support vision health. I find that a lot of people dealing with losing their sight have trouble seeing at night. Bilberry is a good vitamin for night blindness. Studies have shown that supplementation with bilberry improves eye adaptation to darkness for people with poor vision.

If you decide that vitamins are a good choice for you, make sure you do your research, check with your doctor, and find the supplements and foods that will best serve your health needs.

I hope I have been of some help to you in solving problems dealing with your daily health concerns. Just remember, there is only one of you and you are special. YOU must take control of your life and make the effort to stay as healthy as you possibly can. No one can do this except YOU, so get motivated and DO IT!

5

Entertainment and You

∾

Life does not stop just because your eyesight is failing. There are so many fun things for us to do and we can enjoy them just as much as our sighted friends. I love to read, watch a great movie, go to concerts and plays, have a thrilling time at an amusement park, and much, much more. In this chapter, I am going to provide lots of good information and tips that will help you enjoy yourself to the fullest by doing things you thought you could no longer do. Come with me and let's start having fun again!

Reading

Reading is one of my passions. I absolutely love to get lost in the chapters of a good book. I usually have an audio book playing when I am cooking a meal, cleaning my home, or when I want to relax. When I am waiting at the doctor's office a good book sure helps the time fly. With the small, portable devices available today, you can take your book virtually anywhere you need to go.

Did you know that you can get audio books for free? Well, you certainly can! The Library of Congress provides a wonderful talking book program where all materials are delivered to your home via US mail and you simply return them the same way. This service, including all postage, is free to qualifying individuals throughout the United States.

In the early 1930s, the American Foundation for the Blind's (AFB) Talking Books department pioneered the development of recorded books for people who were blind or visually-challenged. Since then, AFB has recorded tens of thousands of books—from textbooks and classic literature to bestsellers and children's books. These books are made available through a provision in the U.S. copyright law and with additional permission granted by the authors and publishers whose works are not specifically covered by this provision. Each year, the National Library Service selects hundreds of books and dozens of magazines and makes them available in a special cassette format that can only be played on specific machines provided by the agency to qualified participants.

Anyone who is unable to access traditional printed material due to either a visual or physical disability can qualify to receive materials through this service. For more information, call the

Help Me! I Am Losing My Sight!

National Library Service at 1-800-424-8567 and they can assist you in contacting the library service in your specific state.

After you get set up with your state's National Library for the Blind and Physically Handicapped and receive your library card number, you can go online and start downloading audio books via the Internet for free. Most of our states' libraries have websites that their patrons can access and download books directly to their computers. You can enjoy listening to all different kinds of books from children's selections, best sellers, classics, and even old time radio shows. You can transfer your selection to a portable device such as an iPod, mp3 player or smart phone which enables you to enjoy your book anywhere you need to go.

The National Library Service now offers a new digital player that is lighter, smaller, and has the capacity to hold more than one book on its cartridges. This unit also has an insert on its side which enables you to download books on to a flash drive. Just log onto your particular library's website or call to find out which downloads are available. If you are interested in this model, or need an upgrade from the four-sided cassette player, call the NLS for more information. Their direct phone number is 202-707-5100.

Do not forget about your own public libraries because they have a great selection of books available on audio. If your local library does not have the one you are interested in reading, check with the librarian who may be able to order it from another location. If you have a smart device, such as a phone or tablet, most public libraries provide an app that will allow you to download books via the Internet.

Another fabulous service that is furnished by The National Federation of the Blind is called the NFB-NEWS LINE. This service provides access to audio versions of hundreds of local and national newspapers and magazines, including weekly sale flyers from stores such as Target. You can also get daily TV guide information, and much, much more. This service is available through your touch-tone phone or the Internet. All services are free to qualifying individuals and application forms can be obtained from the National Federation of the Blind or your state's National Library for the Blind and Physically Handicapped. NFB-NEWS LINE staff can be reached by calling 1-866-504-7300.

If you have a computer and want to read your local newspaper or a newspaper from a neighboring town, you can find it on the Internet. All you have to do is go to your newspaper's website and you can read the paper for free or for a nominal charge.

The American Council of the Blind provides another great Internet option which is the ACB Radio Network. This network delivers a wide range of news, entertainment, talk, and music programming reflecting the interests and experiences of individuals dealing with a vision problem. In fact, most every host is either blind or visually challenged. This programming is delivered free through the Internet and includes the software needed to play it. Visit www.ACBRadio.org and follow the instructions there.

If you do not have a computer, you can also listen to ACB Radio with your phone by calling 231-460-1047. Make sure you get connected to ACB radio, because you never know what helpful and interesting things you might be missing.

Do you like to shop by catalog or read a great magazine? I used to love to look at the Avon catalog or a great fashion brochure with all the new and exciting styles. Then my eyesight progressed to the point where I was unable to look at the pictures and discern what was on the page. After doing a search on the Internet, I was able to find a service called Home Reader's.

The term "Home Readers" is derived from the paid audio transcribers who work from their own homes to record detailed descriptions of catalogs and cookbooks into digital audio formats. Home Readers was established in 1996 as a non-profit organization by Kathy Eble, who is blind, and her husband Bill.

Home Readers provides catalogs, cookbooks, books, and magazines on the special 4-sided cassettes that are made for players that are supplied to visually impaired and blind individuals free of charge by The Library of Congress. These taped magazines allow us to independently shop for items by listening to the detailed descriptions of every item presented. A number of these catalogs can be ordered free of charge. They offer many great magazines such as: Collectors' Choice, Avon, Land's End, Schwann's, Care-A-Lot (Pet products), and many more. Join their Cookbook Club and you will receive a different book filled with recipes each month.

They also offer subscriptions to a limited number of magazines you might also be interested in reading. Upon request, they will provide a free list of catalogs, cookbooks, and books on tape for you to examine. Contact the Home Reader's service at 1-877-814-7323 to receive all of their information. Home Readers is a great service and truly the gateway to shopping for the visually-challenged.

Movies

I really love to watch a good movie and eat a big tub of buttered popcorn with my honey! As my eyesight worsened, the fun of watching a movie diminished because I would miss some of the important details of the story. Action scenes moved too fast, suspense scenes were filled with shadows, and sometimes I missed a detail simply due to my visual impairment. I found this very frustrating until I found a service called Descriptive Video Service (DVS).

This national service makes television programs, feature films, home videos, DVDs, and other visual media accessible to people who are blind or visually-challenged. DVS provides a descriptive narration of the key visual elements in a program or movie which is then inserted within the natural pauses in the dialogue. This enables low-vision viewers to better understand the story. Key visual elements are those which viewers with vision loss would ordinarily miss and include actions, costumes, gestures, facial expressions, scene changes, and onscreen text.

Descriptions are accessed on TV programs via the Second Audio Program (SAP) option, which is standard on most TVs, DVRs, and VCRs. The DVS service is available on stations such as PBS, Turner Classic Movie Channel, CBS, the Fox network, the Nickelodeon channels, and others.

DVS is part of the Media Access Group at WGBH and was launched nationally in 1990 by the WGBH Educational Foundation. This foundation produces many prime-time public television programs and is a leader in the development of accessible media.

If you have never viewed a descriptive video/DVD, I cannot wait for you to experience a movie this way. You will not want to watch another film unless it has the descriptive service. You can watch a movie or program and know exactly what is happening on the screen. This enables you to follow and enjoy it to its fullest! You can contact the Library of Congress to get information concerning these great videos/DVDs. Make sure you ask about the free service provided by many state libraries that will send these videos/DVDs to you through the mail.

There are also free mail services that charge a one-time fee to cover the cost of a movie if you do not send it back. If you keep your account in good standing, you will receive a new one when you return the one you have watched. Do your research and find the service that best suits your needs and I know you will be watching and enjoying great movies again!

Did you know that in some cities throughout the United States, they actually have the DVS service in movie theaters, IMAX theaters, and museums? Well, WGBH successfully developed two innovative technologies that make it possible to provide closed captions and descriptive narrations for deaf and blind patrons, without the need for special prints or screenings or altering the experience for the general audience in theaters. Collectively these systems are known as Motion Picture Access or MoPix.

DVS Theatrical® delivers descriptive narration via infrared or FM listening systems, enabling blind and visually impaired moviegoers to hear the descriptive narration on headsets without disturbing other audience members. Best of all, you can sit anywhere you want in the theater.

A very disheartening fact is that the DVS services are not available in all theaters for us to enjoy. WGBH is working with all the major studios and exhibitors to encourage them to adopt these technologies and make closed captions and descriptive narrations available for more films on an ongoing basis.

As representatives of the blind population we desperately need to contact the trade organizations that represent theater chains and movie studios – the National Association of Theatre Owners (NATO) and the Motion Picture Association of America (MPAA) – to let them know there is an audience of movie fans eager to enjoy films on the big screen. We should have these wonderful services available in all theaters across our nation, especially in our own home towns. We would like to enjoy a movie, IMAX Theater, or museum just like our sighted friends. Please contact these organizations and let your voice be heard!

Concerts, Casinos, and Cruises

Another fun thing to do is to attend a good musical concert. Prior to the concert, call the ticket agent in charge of the particular venue you are attending and tell them your needs. If your sight allows for it, you can ask for seating closer to the stage. I ask for seating that does not require me to tackle a lot of steps. It is usually dark in the theater and I do not want to misstep and fall. When talking to your agent, explain your special needs, and I know you will be seated where you can most enjoy your venue.

Occasionally, I like to venture to a casino and chance my luck. I do not do this often because I do not like giving them my money, but on occasion I find it very exhilarating and fun to place a few bets on the card games and slot machines. If you are like me and enjoy gambling, the dealers are allowed to help you see your cards. When you sit down at a table, inform the dealer of your handicap, and they will be more than happy to assist you.

If you like the slots, ask an employee of the casino and they will help you find what denomination and type of machine you want to play. If you get tired of a machine, ask the waitress to assist you as there is always one readily available for help or a drink. Also, if you have a computer and the right technology loaded on it, you can gamble for fun or for real on the Internet. Just be careful and make sure you are on a legitimate site. I hope this information enables you to have fun gaming, so have a great time and Good Luck to you!

How about really spreading your wings and booking a wonderful voyage on a luxury ship to an exotic destination? Most of the cruise lines accommodate their guests with disabilities. You can arrange an early boarding tour that will help you with orientation so you can become familiar with the ship before others arrive. The main attractions are usually located on the first three levels and often include: casinos, the main dining rooms, theaters, bars, stores and more. You can request the menus in braille, and of course, elevators and rest rooms are all marked as well. You can even bring guide dogs on some of the more personalized trips. If you select an inside cabin, you might be able to book your adventure for a very good price.

My husband and I took our first cruise a few years ago and it was absolutely fantastic! The staff is well trained, ready and willing to help with anything you need. You are treated like royalty and everything you want is right at your fingertips. Get in touch with your travel agency, tell them your special needs, and book a cruise.

Amusement Parks, Museums, and More

Another great adventure would be to plan an exciting visit to one of the various amusement parks. You can enjoy a day at any of the big theme parks such as Disney, Six Flags, Universal, Busch Gardens, or Sea World to name a few. The Americans with Disabilities Act states that guide dogs must be permitted in all of the parks, and there are kennels available to board your dog for a nominal fee. Many of the exhibits and rides have side doors for guests who cannot wait in long lines and employees who will help you with any guidance or assistance getting on or off of a ride. Many parks will provide discounts to people with disabilities or allow a traveling companion to enter without charge. Accommodations for people who are visually challenged differ from theme park to theme park and it is best to make this request prior to your arrival.

My husband, daughter, and I visited Disney World in Florida and had a terrific time. We were given fast passes that enabled us to get on the rides in a very timely manner. We obtained these passes at the customer service department inside the park. The parks do this for your protection and safety. Thank you so much to all of the fun parks that allow us this fantastic service and consideration that makes our visits to them absolutely wonderful!

Did you know that there are museums, zoos, gardens, and parks that provide sensory exhibitions especially for the visually-challenged? Exhibits are equipped with speakers and or headphones which will help you better understand, and fully experience, what you are viewing. Many museums and zoos also have hands-on displays that allow you to feel what you are encountering. These activities can include various animals that you can pet or a special painting that you can touch. Also, a lot of exhibits use the sense of smell or taste to enrich your experience. This could consist of a beautiful garden filled with fragrant flowers or a special wine-tasting tour. You can find the different places offering these sensory exhibits by checking on the Internet, calling the Chamber of Commerce in the city you are visiting, or contacting the NFB (National Federation of the Blind) or ACB (American Council for the Blind) for more information.

I hope this chapter has shown you that there is still tons of fun for you to experience. There are all kinds of places, activities, and groups that are just waiting for you to come and visit. You never know what new friends might make your acquaintance or what wonderful experiences that might be waiting for you. Do your research and find out what is available in your area and neighboring towns. If you are traveling, make a list of things to visit as you make your way to your destination. You have to get out and experience what life has to offer. Be like a flower, open up, and let your senses be tantalized by all the new and exciting possibilities awaiting you!

6

Activities, Fun, and You

❦

When your vision starts to fail, it becomes increasingly difficult to find social-based activities and games that are interesting, fun, and accessible to us as the visually-challenged population. I know that there are a lot of you thinking that there is nothing available for you to do anymore because of your eyesight. You might be thinking that no one will want to be around someone who is blind because you are too much trouble. Stop being preposterous and get motivated to take your life and fun back! In this chapter, I will give you the information needed to contact the many different organizations, companies, and websites that are just waiting for you to come and have an abundance of fun with them.

Did you know that Erik Weihenmeyer became the first blind man to climb Mount Everest in May of 2001? Jeff Evans and his No Limits team finished 2nd on ABC's Expedition Impossible on its first season in the summer of 2011. More significantly, the

5.1 million national viewing audience of Expedition Impossible saw for themselves that disabled athletes, including those without sight, can participate and excel in any challenge that they put their minds and bodies toward. These are just two of the vast number of individuals that took a chance and successfully fulfilled their dreams. What an inspiration and example they have set for the rest of us.

Now, I am not telling you to go out and climb a mountain or do something that you might be uncomfortable with. What I am telling you is there are a lot of activities that you might not have even considered or that you might have thought you could no longer do. You might have to make some adjustments to compensate for your vision, but don't automatically assume that the games, sports, and hobbies you have always enjoyed are now beyond your reach.

The blind and visually-challenged can still participate in many hobbies and activities, including arts and crafts, amateur radio, computer and Internet, wood working, knitting, crocheting, wrestling, weight lifting, judo, water skiing, cross country skiing, skating, swimming, dancing, fishing, crabbing, canoeing, track and field, bowling, shuffleboard, basketball, baseball, volleyball, pool, biking, hiking, mountain climbing, sailing, camping, golf, scuba diving, windsurfing, horseback riding, and so much more. There are accessible games such as chess, checkers, Monopoly, Scrabble, and all kinds of card games. Many video games are also accessible including Zorkthat, which is considered one of the greatest 80's-style adventure classics. Troopanum is an audio-based arcade game similar to Atari's great Space Invaders. Shades of Doom is a first-person shooter game that is sure to please. There are all kinds of arcade-style games, games of chance, pinball simulations, word games, and more available to choose from. Do your research and find what games you might like to play.

Online Games

Here is a partial listing of the companies and organizations making blind-accessible games for us to enjoy.

- PCS Games (www.pcsgames.net) has a large catalog of games in many genres that offer many levels of sophistication.

- Jim Kitchen Games (http://kitchensinc.jgriffith.com) makes simple and free text-based games.

- GMA Games (www.gmagames.com) offers first person shooters, action/arcade, and military simulation using sophisticated audio support.

- DanZ Games (www.danielzingaro.com) provides puzzles and first-person action games.

- BSC Games (http://blindcomputergames.com) makes action and arcade games.

- Bavisoft (www.bavisoft.com) has developed adventure games using primarily sound effects vs. synthesized speech.

- All in Play (http://allinplay.com) provides online games that the blind can play with their fully sighted friends and family as equals.

- The AGRIP Project (http://agrip.org.uk) is an Open Source project working to make mainstream games more accessible to the blind.

- Accessible Games (www.accessiblegames.biz) is a maker of simple, great, low-cost games.

Some of the above websites will allow you to download a free version or a trial version of their games. This is a good way for you to get a feel of the game and know if you truly like it, especially if you have to purchase it.

Hobbies and Sports

I know that, like me, you have been out with your sighted friends and felt excluded from some of their fun activities. Let me share one of my own experiences of dealing with this very thing. My husband and I enjoy visiting a local, family-oriented bar that has several pool tables, pinball machines, dart boards, a shuffle-board table, and many other amusements. We frequently went with our friends to this establishment and I always watched them play the games. I would have a great time, but secretly I wanted to tackle that shuffleboard table and experience it for myself. This was a case of me wanting to play, but not knowing if I could because of my vision. I knew if I was given the chance, I might just be able to play and even win.

Two of my best friends knew of my great desire, so we con-cocted a plan in which we would go to the bar when it was not busy so I could familiarize myself with the table and game. We did this twice a week for about a month. Roy was my partner, and Matt would observe my technique. With their combined coaching abilities, I was soon able to play. I orientated myself to the table and became pretty darn good. Then it was time for my big debut.

We all went to our favorite place for an evening of fun. Roy and I had decided that we would be partners since we had been playing together in practice. Matt and my husband, Richard, became partners and challenged us to my first game. Now, I am not going to say that I was the best shuffleboard player to begin with, but Roy and I have become a formidable team to beat, winning quite frequently. We still enjoy going out and playing to this day, and we absolutely love to annihilate our opponents.

My experience should encourage you to try something new that you might not have thought you could do. If I had not stepped out of my comfort zone and at least tried to play this game, I would have never known how good I could be and how much fun I would have.

Having a good time is such a crucial part of our lives, so please, try to find something fun that will bring great joy into your life.

Below is a list of some of the organizations and their activities that are available specifically to the blind or visually-challenged. I am so excited for you to take a chance and get in touch with one or more of these groups and start having fun again!

- Sports, Games and Recreation for the Blind and Physically Handicapped.
(http://blindreaders.info/sports.html)

- American Blind Bowling Association. Contact: Judy Refosco at 724-745-5986. Address: 315 N. Main St., Houston, PA 15342. This is a membership group of blind bowlers with over 2,000 participants in the U.S. and Canada.

- Blind Camps runs camps for the blind in the USA and Canada. (www.blindcamps.org)

- Space Camp offers specific programs for students with visual impairments. (www.spacecamp.com)

- United States Braille Chess Association for chess enthusiasts who are blind or visually impaired. (www.americanblindchess.org)

- Handi Hams. Amateur radio and technology for people with disabilities. (www.handiham.org)

- Volunteer Match identifies volunteer activities that can be completed, in whole or in part, via the Internet. (www.volunteermatch.org)

- Blind Golf. Blind and vision impaired golf in the United States and worldwide. (www.blindgolf.com)

- Music by Ear. Music instruction in audio format. Phone: 229-249-0628. Address: 704 Habersham Rd., Valdosta, GA 31602.

- PATH International. Therapeutic horseback riding programs. (www.pathintl.org)

- The Tandem Club of America an international club for tandem bike enthusiasts. (http://tandemclub.org)

- Theater By The Blind. A theater troupe based in New York City performed by visually impaired actors. (www.tbtb.org)

- American Blind Skiing Foundation. Skiing programs for visually impaired children & adults. (www.absf.org)

- Ski For Light. Cross-country skiing benefiting blind, visually-impaired, and mobility-impaired individuals and their guides. (www.sfl.org)

- Blind Sailing International. Blind Sailing International is the governing body for competitive international sailing for persons who are blind or visually impaired. (www.blindsailinginternational.com/)

- American Blind Skiers, Inc. Address: 325 Wilshire Blvd., Santa Monica, CA 90403 Phone: 213-828-5514.

- Handicapped Scuba Association. Opening the sport of scuba diving to people with disabilities. (www.hsascuba.com)

- National Beep Baseball Association. A small beeping sound module inside a normal sized softball lets blind people play the game. (www.nbba.org)

- SABAH. Ice Skating Association for the Blind and Handicapped. (www.sabahinc.org)

- Judo for Blind Athletes. Judo is one of the few competitive sports that the visually impaired athlete can participate in fully without major accommodations. (http://judoinfo.com)

- Goalball – From the USA Goalball site. "Goalball is a highly competitive sport played three-against-three, indoors on a gym floor — primarily by blind and visually impaired athletes." There are too many sites to list here but this is both an amateur and professional sport. (www.goalball.us)

- Disabled Sports USA. This organization runs nationwide sports rehabilitation programs open to anyone with a permanent physical disability, including visual impairments. (www.disabledsportsusa.org)

- Challenge Aspen holds a number of sports related camps throughout the year for people with disabilities. (http://challengeaspen.org)

- U.S. Adaptive Recreation Center is one of the largest adaptive recreation programs of its kind, providing winter and summer opportunities for people with disabilities. (http://usarc.org)

- United States Association of Blind Athletes. Competitive sport activities for the blind. (www.usaba.org)

- British Blind Sport. "Providing Sport and Recreation for Blind and Partially Sighted People." (www.britishblindsport.org.uk)

- The International Blind Sports Federation. (www.ibsasport.org)

- The Alliance for Disabled Sportsmen's Rights is a nonprofit organization that coordinates the efforts of disabled individuals who are working to achieve equal access to all hunting, fishing, and outdoor recreation opportunities throughout the United States. E-mail: Alliance@disabledrights.org. (www.disabledrights.org)

I hope this information has really sparked your curiosity and given you the motivation to start having fun again. Recreation is such a vital part of everyone's life and you do not ever lose the urge to experience a great time!

If you have any questions, contact the organization that has captured your interest. They should be able to answer any inquiries you might have or point you in the right direction for more information finding a group close to your location. Also, the American Foundation for the Blind has all of the addresses listed on their web site. I just listed a few and there are many more that you can find with just a little research.

Remember that life does have an expiration date. We must be fulfilled both spiritually and mentally and it goes hand-in-hand with having fun and being happy.

7

Your Kitchen and You

❦

My motto is: You do not need sight to create a great-tasting meal tonight! I really enjoy cooking and I know this chapter will provide a wealth of information for all of your kitchen endeavors. I have been cooking for a long time and know many techniques and gadgets that make preparing a meal easier, quicker, and very blind-friendly. So, with that, come with me and let's take a closer look at our kitchen.

Lighting and Organization

My very first suggestion would be to make sure your prep area and stove is well-lit. This tip alone will help you immensely if you are not totally without vision. A visor placed on your head will help shade your eyes if the light bothers you.

Secondly, to become a good cook you have to be well-organ

-ized and know where your tools and ingredients are located. This is essential if you want to successfully prepare a meal without a great deal of frustration.

One very important tip is to tell anyone who enters your kitchen not to disrupt the way you have it organized. If something is moved ask them to put it back where they originally found it. This way, you will be able to find what you need the next time you are preparing a meal. When creating a dish, make sure you make a mental note of where you set things down such as a spoon, ingredient, or anything you are working with so you can find it again easily.

I suggest that you keep the ingredients that you are working with close at hand on a tray or baking pan with raised sides. This will keep everything you need contained and at your fingertips.

Labeling your spices is mandatory. You do not want to add red pepper to a dish when it calls for black pepper, as this can create a disaster and ruin the meal you have worked so hard to prepare. Sometimes the shape, size, or feel of a bottle can help you determine what is in it.

I like to buy the big bottles of spices that I use on a daily basis such as salt, garlic powder, red pepper, black pepper, and so on. In this case, I use rubber bands to identify the bottles of spices such as two bands for the garlic powder, four for the red pepper. You can also use raised tactile dots to mark your spice containers. Tactile dots and rubber bands come in different sizes and thicknesses so you can create your own easy-to-find system. If your sight is still relatively good, stick a piece of white duct tape to your bottle and label with a thick, black felt pen. You can use abbreviations such as GP for garlic powder and RP for red pepper. You could also use different colors of lids if you can still distinguish color.

Remember, when you empty a spice container that you have marked, fill it back up so you do not have to label a new bottle. When you are through with a spice, immediately put the lid on it and place it back where you keep it.

In addition to labeling your spices, remember to use your sense of smell. Most spices have a distinctive aroma which will help you identify them. So, don't forget to use your nose.

Your staples, such as canned goods, boxed goods, or items in jars or plastic packaging should be organized to your unique specifications. You can buy divider strips to put in your cabinets and drawers to separate your food items like canned soups, canned tomato products, green beans, etc. If you have a certain section of your cabinet that you always store the different items, although they might look and feel the same, you will know what they are by where they are placed. If you are familiar with Braille, you can use it to label the different sections or, if your sight allows, use a bold felt pen. Do not forget about the bar code reader and the PenFriend as either one of these can be a fantastic help to you in the kitchen. Once again, I am going to remind you to tell everyone that enters your kitchen to leave everything exactly as it was for your own peace of mind.

I like storing my utensils in a big ceramic container such as an old cookie jar or a crock. The container keeps your utensils stored within easy reach and you are not fumbling in a drawer for what you are seeking.

Placing hooks in discreet places around your kitchen will help you find items you reach for frequently. This includes your apron, cooking utensils, measuring cups and spoons, pot holders, or any other thing you need to locate quickly and easily.

One of my main helpers that sits on my counter every single day is a garbage bowl. As I am preparing a recipe, I can discard any trash such as vegetable peelings, food wrappers, or anything that needs thrown away. The right size bowl will enable you to put a bag in it to keep the mess contained so you can easily take it to your bigger trash. This kitchen hint will save you a lot of steps.

Tools and Gadgets

There are innumerable tools and gadgets that are made specifically to enhance our experience in the kitchen. This means that we are able to prepare and cook our recipes much faster and easier if we take advantage of them. Let me tell you about some of my favorites.

My best tool in the kitchen is a good sharp knife. A dull knife is extremely dangerous, because of the extra pressure you use to do a task. Find a good knife that is comfortable in your hand and keep it sharpened. I have a great knife block that I really like. Its design does not have the individual knife slots. Instead, it has thin, flexible, straw-like sticks placed in the block that allow your knife to slide in anywhere and at any position. This block can hold up to 18 knives. You just slide the point of the knife into the block and the knife is stored with only the handle visible. The knife block comes in many styles and is made by a company called Kapoosh. You can find it at their website, www.kapoosh.com.

The main ingredient of a well-stocked kitchen is a quality set of non-stick cookware. The non-stick coating will make cooking your favorite recipes very easy and clean-up a breeze. You can find brands of non-stick cookware that are metal utensil friendly, allowing you to use your metal utensils without damaging the integrity of the pans.

A square shaped skillet is an excellent tool for cooking eggs. Break the egg in the corner and you have the sides as a guide to pick it up or turn it over. A thin edge spatula is the best for getting under the egg. Over easy, please!

The appliance I really enjoy using is an electric skillet because it can have a larger cooking area, the temperature is easy to control, and it is very stable on a counter top. If you are interested in purchasing one, make sure it has non-skid bottoms on its feet. You can easily mark the temperature control with raised tactile dots. I like to put one on 350 degrees, because I can gauge my temperature setting whether it is above or below this dot. Also, make sure the skillet is non-stick for easy cleaning.

A deep fryer is a great tool to prepare many types of fun and tasty foods. When selecting a deep fryer, make sure it has a stay-cool exterior and a raise and lower knob for the basket. The temperature control should be marked with a raised tactile dot at 370 degrees for optimum frying. When the oil is at the right temperature, the outside of your food sears quickly, and you can fry healthier. Be sure to dry your food well with paper towels before adding it to the grease. This will reduce splattering and help you avoid burns. Each food item that you prepare will have a certain frying time, and a talking timer is a great item to accompany your fryer. Likewise, a talking kitchen thermometer is handy for checking the temperature of your oil, the doneness of all kinds of meat, and so much more. This thermometer will also alleviate any fear of getting sick from undercooked food.

Did you know that there are talking microwaves? I love anything that speaks to me, but many of these appliances can be very costly. I suggest that you mark a traditional microwave with raised tactile dots at your preferred settings. This could be on the popcorn setting, defrost function, or especially the minute button. You can actually prepare a great tasting, healthy meal with the right microwave safe cookware. There are steamers, rice cookers, grilling pans, pressure cookers, and many more that will help you with your meal preparation. You can use them very easily and they can save you a great deal of time.

A huge break-through that has benefited the blind cook is the invention of silicone. There are all shapes and sizes of bake ware made out of this amazing material. It cools rapidly, cleans easily and it will not rust or dent. You do not need to spray the surface of silicone with cooking spray because it is naturally non-stick.

A silicone baking board is great when placed in the bottom of your oven to keep it clean. The board will catch any spill over messes from your pans during baking. If a spill over occurs, just remove the silicone baking board, clean it, and return it to the oven. These boards are also great for making cookies or a yummy pile of French fried potatoes covered in cheese.

The cookies and cheesy French fries will slide right off for easy clean up.

Invest in cooking utensils with silicone handles because they will not get hot and you can avoid a burn. I found a set of stainless steel utensils that are unique in the way they have a design-bend in the handle. This allows them to hang securely on the inside of your pan which eliminates the need for a spoon rest. The lid still fits on your pan and the silicone handle is easily accessible. You can find these utensils in many stores and online under Lori Greiner or Rachel Ray's products.

Other great silicone items include:

- Flexible cutting boards. After you prepare your ingredients for your recipe you can bend the board in half making it so easy to add them to your dish.

- Basting brushes. This is great when cooking on the grill, because it is flame retardant and will not catch on fire.

- Aprons and gloves. You can purchase gloves with five finger slots for easy gripping. The apron is also waterproof, so when washing dishes or bathing your dog you will stay comfortably dry.

- Oven rack guards. These fit on the very front of the oven racks so there aren't any accidental burns.

- Bowls, colanders, and measuring cups. I love these because they are flexible and can collapse flat for easy storage.

- Universal lids for your cookware. These are great because one lid fits different sizes of pans. No more searching for the right sized lid!

Silicone is truly a blind cook's blessing. It is just so exciting that a product can do so many things and protect us as well. Check online and in your local kitchen stores for all of your choices made with silicone.

You need to have a good set of measuring cups and spoons in your collection of kitchen tools. They have cups that are stacked in order from one cup to one-fourth cup. These measuring cups are usually made of ceramic and stack to form a design such as an apple, pear, Christmas tree, and more. This makes it easy to identify each of your measuring cups, because they are stacked in order ranging from the largest amount to the smallest.

I suggest getting a four-sided measuring spoon, because it has all of the common measurements in an all-in-one utensil which makes it easy to use and saves space. You can also identify your measuring cups and spoons by color if your vision allows for this. You can purchase these measuring cups and spoons where each utensil has its own specific color.

Another favorite tool of mine is a food processor, because this device can literally cut your time in half when making a recipe. It is very easy to label your settings with raised tactile dots. Put one on stop and one on process. Vegetables, fruits, meats, cheeses, and nuts can all be sliced and chopped easily and efficiently. Make sure that you do not remove the lid until the unit has come to a complete stop as you do not want any finger tips in your recipe!

A crock pot is also a wonderful tool for our blind kitchen. You can put all of your ingredients in it in the morning and your meal will be ready in the evening. You are able to prepare healthy meals for your family in just one pot and it will be ready for you when you return home from work or play.

Another fantastic kitchen appliance is a George Foreman Grill. It reduces fat as it cooks the food on both sides at once. This allows you to quickly and easily grill all types of meats, vegetables, and fruits in a very timely manner. If your grill does not have the removable plates, here is a great tip: After you are finished grilling with your George Foreman, unplug it and place a damp dish towel in-between the top and bottom grill plates while they are still hot. Let it sit for about five minutes, and this will help loosen any mess on the plates for easy cleanup.

Another outstanding gadget I use on a regular basis is an onion chopper. I have one that has the cup attached to it, making it easy to catch the chopped onion and add it to my dish. All you have to do is peel your onion and cut it in half, place it on the marked raised surface, and push the top down hard and fast. This produces great pieces of chopped onions. You can also chop other types of veggies and fruits with this as well. The Nicer Dicer and Genius are two great brands available.

The very best tool you can use in the kitchen is your own two hands. Make sure you wash them thoroughly before you dig in to that special recipe. Use your hands to rub seasonings in to meats, poultry, pork, and seafood as this will help the flavor envelop the food. Also, your palms can be used to measure spices easily. The sense of touch is one of our great assets, so use it!

If you never want the embarrassment of over filling a cup or glass again, I suggest you obtain a beverage indicator. Place the device on the side of your container, and when the desired level is reached, the indicator will beep so you will know when it is full. This gadget is particularly useful for hot liquids, because you will no longer have the fear of scalding yourself. When filling your own glass, you can discreetly place your finger inside the top of it and fill it until the liquid touches your fingertip. Use this suggestion at your own personal discretion.

Sometimes it is hard to locate a glass after you have set it down, because the glass could be clear and filled with ice water, making it very difficult to see. You do not want to knock it over and embarrass yourself, especially if you are in public. I find that if I use my knife as a pointer, and place the glass at its tip, the knife will always be pointing to my drink where I can easily find it.

General Safety Techniques

The most important kitchen tip I can stress to you in this chapter is to try and be safe in everything you do. Think about things before you do them and plan ahead for any unforeseen contingency. I know this is not possible in all scenarios, but at times it can really be a blessing. Try to be aware of your surroundings with all of your senses whether it is your vision, hearing, touch, or smell.

One contingency plan is to keep a fire extinguisher and a container of baking soda within easy reach of your cooking area. Do not ever use water or flour to put out a fire, because this can make it spread quickly. Learn to use your fire extinguisher before an emergency occurs. If you are not sure about a situation, get your family and yourself safely out of harm's way.

Help Me! I Am Losing My Sight!

Meanwhile back in our safe kitchen:

- Avoid a grease buildup on your stove by cleaning it after every meal.

- Do not leave the house if food is simmering, baking or roasting.

- Never leave cooking food unattended on the stove.

- If you have any length to your hair, make sure it is pulled back in a ponytail or contained in a hat or scarf.

- Do not wear clothing that drapes or hangs.

- Make sure kitchen towels and potholders are located away from your cooking surface.

- Turn your pot handles inward, so you do not accidentally knock your pan off of the stove.

- If you are unsure of a food item, throw it out.

- Keep your oven, pantry, and cabinet doors closed to keep from running into them and hurting yourself.

Remember, safety first in everything we do!

General Cooking Tips

I would like to share a few tips that I have learned and use on a daily basis to make my own experience in the kitchen fun, easy, and quick.

I really like using bacon as an ingredient or by itself. A good way to prepare it is to use a large enough baking pan to place it side-by-side allowing it to lay flat. Bake at 380 degrees until your desired crispiness is reached, about 25 minutes. You do not have to turn the bacon over, making it very blind friendly to prepare. All ovens do not cook the same, so use your sense of smell to determine when it is done.

An easy way to peel a boiled potato is to place them in cool water after cooking. This will lower the temperature making it easy to pick them up. Then, place the potato inside a clean dish towel and simply rub the outer skin off. This makes it quite easy to peel and also contain the mess.

To make your own self-rising flour, add 1 1/2 teaspoons baking powder and 1/2 teaspoon salt to 1 cup all-purpose flour. Make as much as you need and you can store the extra in an air-tight container.

An easy way to remove sour cream, condensed soup, tomato paste, and other products of this consistency is to turn the container over and punch a hole in the bottom. After this is accomplished, turn the container back over and open it. Now, place your lips over the hole and blow. Make sure your ingredient is over a bowl, because the product will slip out of its container very easily.

For peeling peaches and tomatoes quickly, mark an "X" on one end with a sharp knife, drop them in some boiling water for two to four minutes and then transfer them to a bowl of ice water right away. The skin should just slide right off.

Remember, when using rice, keep in mind that 1 cup of uncooked long-grain white rice will make 3 cups cooked. So gauge your meal accordingly.

Instead of the water your recipe calls for, try chicken broth or a type of juice for more flavor.

To select the freshest eggs, open the egg carton and feel the shells. Fresh eggs are rough and chalky; old eggs are smooth and shiny.

When separating an egg, crack the egg into your hand and let the white of the egg run through your fingers, leaving the yolk of the egg remaining in your palm.

Make no-mess pancakes with the help of a ketchup bottle. This will allow you to squeeze out precise portions of batter and form the perfect breakfast treat. Be sure to label your bottle, store it in the refrigerator, and do not keep the batter for more than three days.

Microwave a lemon or lime about 20 seconds to produce more juice.

If you need garlic for a recipe, microwave the cloves for 15 seconds and the skins should slip right off.

Thaw fish in milk for a fresher flavor and no fishy taste will occur.

For a more succulent flavor when grilling meat or poultry, let it rest for at least five minutes after you remove it from the grill.

When buying a bag of potatoes, place an apple in it to prevent the eyes from growing and your potatoes will last longer.

To pick a sweet pineapple, pull off a leaf and if it releases easily, it is ripe and ready to eat.

The best way to store fresh celery is to wrap it in aluminum foil, put it in the refrigerator, and it will keep for weeks.

Place your tomatoes stem side down and they will stay fresher longer.

Help Me! I Am Losing My Sight!

After shucking fresh corn, a dampened paper towel or dish cloth brushed downward on the cob of corn will help remove every strand of silk.

Noodles, spaghetti and other starches will not boil over if you rub the inside of the pot with vegetable oil.

When filling a container, place your hand against the side of it near the top. This should allow you to feel the difference in temperature between the liquid and container as it reaches the fill line. Also, the distinct sound of the liquid as it reaches the top can be easily heard and controlled with practice.

For perfect boiled eggs, place them in a pan filled with cold water. Make sure the water covers the eggs thoroughly. Bring the water to a boil, place a lid on it, and turn the heat off. Let the eggs stand in the hot water for about 10 minutes. After the minutes have elapsed, transfer the eggs to the sink and run cold water over them to reduce the heat. Then, crack the egg and hold it under lightly running water to easily peel.

To gauge when the water is boiling in a pan, place your hand on the handle or lid to feel the rolling action of the water. Make sure to use your silicone gloves or a pot holder to avoid a burn.

When preparing corn on the cob, add 2 heaping tablespoons

of sugar or 1 heaping tablespoon of Splenda to the water to add sweetness to the corn.

If you ever have problems with ants in your kitchen, buy some clove spice and sprinkle it where you suspect the ants are coming in. Not only will the ants leave, you will have a pleasant fragrance in your kitchen.

One last tip that I find very useful is this: if you happen to get a splinter in your skin, squeeze a generous amount of Elmer's glue over the area, let it dry thoroughly, and peel the dried glue from the location. The splinter should adhere to the dried glue and come right out.

I sincerely hope that this information concerning your kitchen has given you the courage and inspiration to try something new. You must take baby steps until you are feeling comfortable in your cooking environment. The love expressed in the preparation of a great dish nurtures the mind, body, and soul, making our kitchens the most important location in our homes.

Here is one of my own recipe creations and it is a real crowd pleaser. Enjoy!

Nonie's Scrumptious Taco Soup

Garnishing ingredients:
  Sliced jalapenos
  Chopped green onions
  Grated cheese
  Sour cream
  Corn chips

Cooking ingredients:
  1- 1-ounce package Hidden Valley ranch salad dressing mix
  1- 1 1/4-ounce package McCormick's taco seasoning mix original
  3 heaping tablespoons sugar or substitute 2 heaping tablespoons Splenda
  2- 4 1/2-ounce cans diced green chilies or fresh chilies
  1 can diced black olives optional
  1- 28 oz. can diced tomatoes
  1- 10 ounce can Rotel tomatoes with chilies original
  1- 10 ounce can tomatoes Rotel hot, or if you do not want it to be hot add another can of original or mild instead
  1- 10 oz. can Rotel tomato chili fixings
  3- 14 oz. cans of chicken broth
  2- 15 1/4-ounces cans whole kernel corn, drained
  1- 15-1/2 ounce can pinto beans
  2 cups diced onions
  3 to 4 lbs. ground beef or chili meat

Directions:

Brown the ground beef and onions in a large skillet; drain the excess fat, then transfer the browned beef and onions to a large Crockpot or a stockpot. Add the beans, corn, tomatoes, broth, chilies, olives, and seasonings, and cook on a low setting all day (6 to 8 hours) if using a Crockpot, or simmer over low heat for about 1 to 2 hours in a stockpot on the stove.

To serve, place a few corn chips in each bowl and ladle soup over them. Top with sour cream, cheese, green onions, and jalapeños if desired.

Servings: 12 to 16 servings

Prep Time: 15 min

Cook Time: 8 hours crock pot; 1 to 2 hours stock pot

Difficulty: Easy

This soup freezes easily, so you can make individual servings for later if you like.

8

Your Home and You

✍

Whether you can see or not, I do not think anyone really enjoys cleaning; it is simply a necessity that we have to endure. If you can afford a housekeeping service, congratulations! But sadly, if you are like me, you will have to become your own domestic engineer. With that in mind, I have gathered here my best strategies to help you keep your home clean, safe, and enjoyable.

Cleaning

Before you begin, you must decide that a clean home is important to you. This determination will give you the incentive to start tackling your living space one issue at a time. Once everything is done to your satisfaction, make sure you try to maintain what you have accomplished. This will ultimately save you a lot of time and frustration.

The first tip I suggest is to try and keep your rooms and furniture clutter-free. This will reduce your chances of knocking over or breaking something dear to you. Think about what treasures you would really like to put on display and make a mental note of where they are located. Less clutter makes it easier and quicker to keep things clean and in order.

Every room in your home will not need to be cleaned every week. For instance, a guest bedroom will not need your attention as often as a high-traffic area.

I suggest breaking your living space into sections as you clean. Do one job at a time, such as dusting, sweeping, or mopping. All of these task can be quickly and efficiently accomplished by using tools made from microfiber. Microfiber is a great option because it is capable of absorbing up to seven times its own weight in moisture and can be used safely on any surface. It easily captures dirt, dust, and most liquids. Since microfiber leaves less moisture on a surface, there is less chance of bacteria growth, leaving your home environment healthier. To clean: Wash and dry them by themselves and do not use bleach or fabric softener. This tip will keep your tools in a good usable condition for a longer period of time.

When you get ready to dust, I suggest using a microfiber glove. It literally attracts dust like a magnet, making this job both fast and effective. Put one glove on one hand and leave the other hand gloveless to serve as a guide. This way the gloved hand can follow behind the gloveless hand and you will not be afraid of accidentally damaging one of your treasures.

Vacuuming can be a really cumbersome chore which is best done later. This reason is why I took my time and researched many vacuum cleaners before I decided to invest in a Roomba. After seeing it work on my own floors, I absolutely fell in love. You never have to push around a vacuum cleaner again, because this is a robot. The Roomba picks up dirt, dust, hair, crumbs, and other debris as it independently navigates throughout your home. This robot automatically adjusts from carpets to hard floors and cleans everywhere you want while avoiding off-limit areas. It cleans under your furniture and does not get tangled in your wires.

I really like this vacuum, especially because I can set it and forget it while it cleans. Everyone is amazed at the dirt and debris it picks up. There are other kinds of robots available that will mop your floors, maintain your pool, clean your gutters, and more. To find out about these robots, you can contact the i-Robot Corporation directly at 1-800-727-9077 with any questions.

If you are cleaning with a broom, break your area into four sections. Place an unused toilet plunger in the middle of your room and this will serve as a guide to sweep towards. You can purchase them in different colors to make a strong visual contrast, enabling you to see it better. As you begin to clean your floor, start in a corner and sweep towards the plunger. Make sure you use a method that allows you to overlap the broom stroke you have just made. When you have covered your entire surface and swept the debris to the middle, get your dust pan, remove the plunger, and sweep the mess into the pan. Then, discard it into the trash. I like to use a plunger because it has a long handle, is lightweight and easy to move, and serves well as a marker.

Use this same method when mopping and vacuuming minus the plunger. Make sure you overlap the swipe you have just made and you will be able to easily cover and clean your entire floor.

Another great tip is to keep all of your cleaning supplies together and organized in a lightweight caddie with a handle so you will know where they are located. This will make it easy to take your tools from room to room as you clean.

I love walking into my home and being enveloped in a wonderful scent, such as sweet-smelling potpourri, a scented candle, or a fragrant plug-in. However, if you are dealing with a bad smell that lingers, I suggest you use vinegar to eliminate it. Pour white vinegar into a bowl and place it in discreet locations around your home. This simple tip will get rid of most hardcore odors. Check the bowls every few days to clean or refill them.

Baking soda is also a very good option to deter unpleasant smells. Sprinkle some in your trash and cat litter and place a box in your refrigerator and freezer.

To keep your garbage disposal clean and odor-free, pour ½ cup of baking soda followed by 1 cup of vinegar into it. Listen for the bubble and fizz and let this concoction sit and work for five to ten minutes. Then pour a few cups of boiling water down the disposal to wash away the remaining residue and leave your drain smelling good. You can also create a pleasant scent by putting citrus rinds, such as oranges, lemons, or limes, down the disposal along with a few ice cubes. Turn your disposal on for a few minutes and let the ice cubes sharpen the blades and remove any excess debris caused by the rinds.

A quick way to take care of your bathroom is to pour two cups vinegar and sprinkle one-half cup baking soda in your toilet bowl. While it is fizzing, get some disinfecting wipes and clean your vanity and tub. Use your microfiber towel to wipe down your mirror and fixtures. Grab your toilet brush to thoroughly clean the toilet and finish up with disinfecting wipes on the seat, tank, and handle. Put a little disinfecting spray on your microfiber towel and while backing out of your bathroom, use your foot on the towel to clean your floor. Do not forget to empty your trash. Bathroom is done!

Another important room in your home is the kitchen. It is considered the very heart and hub of your home, so keep it clean and looking good.

Here are a few strategies to accomplish this:

- Your sink and counter tops are the main focal points of your kitchen, so keep them clean and clutter-free.

- Dry your sink with paper towels to make it shine.

- A small hand-held vacuum is a great tool for cleaning counter tops and floors around your prep area.

- Clean your stove after every use to avoid a grease build-up.

- Use a small amount of baby or olive oil on a microfiber towel to clean and wipe away fingerprints on your stainless steel appliances.

- Wipe down your cabinets once a week to keep them looking great.

- Clean and disinfect your doorknobs, keyboards, phone, light switches, and anything else that comes in contact with hands.

My best advice for your kitchen is to form a good maintenance plan and stick to it.

As for your master bedroom, I am sure your mother told you to make your bed every day when you were growing up. Your bed is the primary focal point of your room, so follow your mother's advice and keep it made and looking good. Pick all of your clothes and shoes up from the floor. Organize them in your closet with your own special system. Follow the simple rule of "taking something out and then putting it right back" and you will be able to find everything easily. Make sure all of your drawers are shut so you do not accidentally run in to them and hurt yourself. Take a few minutes each day to put everything where it belongs and your room will become a warm, welcoming environment allowing you to relax when it is time to go to bed.

Other Tips and Tools

A great source of lighting for your outside living space is a solar powered option. Solar lights are very décor-friendly, inexpensive, and are powered by only the sun. Place them around your walkway and the entrance to your home to serve as a beacon. They will help you determine where you need to walk and exactly where your door is located after dark.

If you have stairs that lead to your door, invest in brightly colored or glow-in-the-dark tape strips. Apply them directly to the edge of each step to make them more visible.

One suggestion for your mail box is to place a solar light by it if you collect your mail after the sun goes down. This will help you find it, especially when the days are shorter in the winter. A light alert is another nifty device used in conjunction with your post box. Place the sensor in your box and the receiver in your home and when your mail carrier deposits your mail, you will be alerted via sound and light.

Another great suggestion is to invest in a talking thermostat for your central air. This will enable you to set your own personal comfort level without help. It could also save you money on your monthly bill, because you can keep a closer eye on the temperature.

Did you know that there is scientific proof that the act of cleaning has many physical, mental, and emotional benefits that may improve our health? This fact alone should encourage you to start planning a good regimen of cleaning. The hardest part is to get started, but after you finish, it is very rewarding to have a clean, fresh-smelling home that you can be extremely proud of.

9

Personal Care and You

❧

It may not be possible for you to see yourself clearly in a mirror, but please do not use this as an excuse to neglect your appearance. You might think that nobody is concerned about the way you look and maybe you are correct. But, in my humble opinion, you should be the only one who recognizes that it is indeed important. Your body is a reflection of your inner self, so making positive changes will facilitate good confidence and bring forth many beneficial results. You will find yourself standing a little taller and your persona will shine so much brighter.

Did you know that everyone has their own unique voice, fingerprints, and DNA profile that is strictly theirs alone? So, the next time you are feeling imperfect think about how extremely special you truly are. There is no one else in this world that is just like you, and you are exceptional.

Getting Started

The first thing I would like to do is to remind you that maintaining a good regimen of personal hygiene is very important. This includes washing your hands, brushing and flossing your teeth, and generally keeping yourself clean and presentable. Practicing good body hygiene is essential and will ultimately keep you feeling very confident.

When you get dressed, use your color identifier discussed in Chapter Three to determine the color of your clothes and accessories. Try to wear clothes that are comfortable and in style. Do not wear a shirt that makes you feel self-conscious or a pair of pants that are way too tight. Choose clothing that will enhance your attributes such as hair, eye, and skin color. Make a date with one of your sighted friends or family members and go shopping for something new. They can help you determine what styles are flattering.

Organize your closet by hanging your garments together in a color-coded system. Place all of your reds in one group, your blacks in another, and so on. You can also identify your clothes by touch. In some cases, the fabrics are different and you can tell which item is which is by feel. The bar code reader and Pen-Friend are also great tools for identification if you have labeled your things. If all else fails, ask a sighted person to help you coordinate your outfits and hang them together.

Make sure shoes are stored with their matching mate for quick identification. I am one of those shoppers that when I find a comfortable, good-looking pair of shoes, I might buy more than one pair of the same style. One day I was at the mall with one of my friends when they looked down and noticed that I had on two different colors of shoe. It was not that obvious, because the color was black and navy in the same style. This taught me an important lesson of making sure my shoes match before I leave home. When you are dressed and feel good about your appearance, your self-assurance will blossom!

Applying Makeup

The art of applying makeup should be fun and trouble-free, but when your vision starts to fail the process can be difficult. I know since my own eyesight has declined, I have had to master a few issues myself. The use of makeup is strictly a personal choice and it is up to your discretion if you want to use it or not. But, if you are interested and want to know more, I am going to share a few tips I have learned over the years

First Steps

Before you can apply makeup, you have to take the time to

get really familiar with your face. You will need to meticulously study and learn every line, angle and contour of every section by using your fingertips. For example, if you touch your lips you can definitely feel the outline of them. Your jawline has a definite angle, as do your cheek bones. Get acquainted with your eyelashes, brows, and general eye area. You can feel where your eyebrow arches and, further up, your hairline begins. When you get completely familiar and comfortable with every part of your face, you will then be able to apply makeup.

Suggestions before starting:

- Play with your makeup like a newbie until you get the hang of it and its application. All makeup brands do wash off so you can practice applying it as many times as you like. Remember, practice makes perfect.

- Store your daytime and evening makeup products separately, including all coordinating colors.

- Mark your pencils and other makeup with rubber bands, stick-on markers, a felt pen, or use your bar code reader or PenFriend for identification.

- Keep your products in the refrigerator for a definite temperature difference when you are applying them.

- Apply your makeup using a light touch as you do not want it to appear clownish.

- Blend your products thoroughly for a natural look that closely matches your skin-tone.

I have passed the point of being able to see myself clearly in a mirror so I do not use one when applying my makeup. I do not need one because I am very familiar with my own face. My friends and family members are astonished when they see me applying my products without looking. The only thing I strongly suggest is to ask a buddy if you look okay after you are finished.

One day, I was leaving with a friend to go to an appointment. He took one look at me and started laughing out loud. I was perplexed as to why he was laughing so hard so I asked him what was wrong. He pointed at my lips and questioned if I had intended to wear a green lip color. I started laughing too, and I told him that I thought green lips were the current style. The truth was that I had applied a mood matching lip color that was out of date and it did not change to the pink color it should have. This episode is a great reminder to ask a sighted person to check your makeup application. You do not want to have a black eye due to mascara, or bright green lips like I did.

A great tip is to schedule a free makeup appointment at a high-end department store, such as Macy's, Dillard's, or another similar retailer. These stores have a selection of different name-brand counters where professional face artists can help you learn how to apply their products and find the colors best suited to your skin tone. This is a great idea, because you can feel exactly where she is applying each item and you can voice any question or concern as it happens. Take a pad of paper and pen with you to your appointment so the artist can write down the products she used, and their colors, for future reference. Also, if possible have her place some of the color right on your pad for a better color-match, so if you cannot afford the products at these stores, you can purchase something similar elsewhere.

Specific Makeup Techniques

Remember, it is important to wash your hands every time you touch your makeup, so you do not cross-contaminate your products or face.

Now, grab your makeup bag and let's begin. We are going for a natural look. Pull your hair back away from your face. Make sure your skin is thoroughly cleansed and ready. Next, use a good moisturizer and let it completely absorb into your skin. I like to start with my eyes in case I accidentally get mascara on my face during the application. If I have a mascara mishap, I can easily clean the area without also removing any other makeup on my skin.

Starting with your eyes, use an easy-glide eyeliner pencil to line your eyes. Hold the pencil as close to the point-end as you can, as this will help you with stability and control. Place the pointer finger of your opposite hand on your eyelid to show where your lash line is located. Line only the outer two-thirds of your eye. Leaving a space unlined on the inside corners gives a softer, less severe look.

If you are older, you might want to make the line a little thicker and lift it up a touch on the outer corner of the upper lid. This creates a lift-illusion. Make sure you draw the line on the lower lashes to the very end, connecting the upper and bottom lines at the outer corner. Finally, lightly smudge.

Use your eyelash curler and curl your eyelashes. If you are unable to apply mascara one-handed with just the wand, you can control the applicator by placing your pointer finger on the end of the brush-side. Use your thumb as an anchor on your cheek, close to the corner of your mouth. Bring the brush slowly to your lashes until you can feel your lashes connect with it as you blink. I only coat the top lashes, because it is too hard for me to do the bottom and not make a mess. Blink your eye lashes against the applicator to build and define.

If you would like to get rid of any unwanted clumps of mascara and finish separating your lashes, use a soft toothbrush. Purchase a new one and use it only for this purpose. Use your eyelash curler again to really enhance your lashes, especially for an evening look.

Now it is time to apply foundation and remember: a little goes a long way. You can also use a tinted moisturizer for a daytime look. If you keep your makeup in the refrigerator, you will be able to tell exactly where you are applying it. Make sure you cover your entire face and blend well. Because we are going for a natural look and not using eye shadow, put a teeny, tiny amount of it on your eyelids to match the rest of your face.

Use a wet Q-tip to clean your eyebrows. Place your pointer finger of the hand that is not holding the Q-tip to the outer edge of your brow. Rub it backwards towards your nose following the hair. You will feel the definite outline of your eyebrows. Now trace and clean the brow with the Q-tip following your pointer finger.

Use an eyebrow pencil with the same method, placing your fingers as close to the application end of the pencil as possible. Lightly add the color, feeling for the hairs and outer edge of your brows. If you do not like applying eyebrow pencil, do what I do, and get your brows dyed at the beauty salon. You only have to do this about three to four times a year and you will never worry about applying the eyebrow pencil again.

Smile real big and you will be able to tell where the apples of your cheeks are located. Add a little blush on your brush and swipe upward toward your ear, starting in the center of your cheek and following the bone. Now blend. Do not get the blush close to your hairline, because you do not want the color to intermix with your hair. You know me; I experienced this before and was told in public that I had pink tinges in my hair. I told that particular person that I was going for a punk-rocker look. How inwardly embarrassing!

Now it is time to focus on our lips. I like to use an applicator that has a definite edge such as a wand or brush. Any applicator with an edge will help you stay in the confines of your lips, because you can feel where the color is being applied. Also, again, if your cosmetics are fresh out of the refrigerator, you will feel a definite temperature difference.

As you are applying your lip product, place your little finger on your chin for support and stability. When you are finished, press your lips together and rub them back and forth to thoroughly coat them with color. Next, place your pointer finger between your top and bottom lips and slowly pull your finger out of your mouth pressing your lips together around your finger. The excess product that would have been on your teeth will now be on your finger. This beauty hint will keep you smiling with no fear of color on your teeth. I have been very frustrated and embarrassed to learn after I have walked around in public that I had been smiling at people with lipstick on my teeth. Use this hint: wipe the front of your teeth with a Kleenex for extra protection against this happening.

Your makeup is done and I know you look gorgeous!

If you have a problem applying eyeliner, I suggest getting your liner permanently done by an aesthetician. I chose this option for myself, because as my eyesight diminished, I could never get it applied correctly. I got tired of my liner being uneven, especially on the lower lash-line, so getting my eyelids tattooed has been a great choice for me. I am not telling you personally to get your eyes done, but it is an option that I thought you should be aware of. You also have the option of getting a permanent color on your lips or eyebrows. If you decide to take the plunge, make sure you get a reputable aesthetician with good reviews from their former clients.

My final makeup tip is to view makeup application videos on YouTube. It is a wealth of information on makeup contouring and application just waiting for you to visit.

Healthy Skin

Did you know that your skin is the biggest organ in your body? It is imperative that we take care of it by doing the following:

- Wear a hat and use products with a good sun screen anytime you are going to be outside. The sun increases your risk for developing skin cancer and actually accelerates the effects of aging.

- Wear sunglasses to stop premature aging around your eyes and prevent sun damage to the corneas. The sun is one of the culprits that cause cataracts.

- Cleanse and moisturize your skin every day to prevent clogged pores resulting in breakouts. It is scientifically documented that taking care of your skin has many benefits, so find what products work for you.

- Exfoliate your face and body at least once a week to get rid of dry, dead skin. This will ultimately help improve the results of your skin care and bring new life to your complexion.

- Label your products. This will insure that you definitely know what is in your hand before application.

I made the mistake of not following this important tip, and ended up with an unexpected mishap. One night as I lay in my bed, I noticed that my face felt very dry. I reached into my bedside table drawer and pulled out a jar of what I thought was my face cream. I generously applied it to my face to relieve the dryness. After about two minutes of this cream soaking into my skin, I started to feel a temperature difference. My face became warm, and still warmer as I lay there. It started to become hot so I hurried to the bathroom and quickly cleaned my face. I washed and rinsed my face at least three times before the burning began to subside. I then, applied a generous amount of my true face cream and went back to bed with a cold cloth to soothe my skin.

The next morning, I ask my husband what in the world did I put on my face last night. We went to the bedside table and pulled out a container of KY warming jelly. I had only tried this one time and did not care for it, so it was left in the drawer without another thought. This time I threw it directly in the trash and we both had a side-splitting laugh over my mishap! It always seems that I have to learn everything the hard way and this was a painful reminder to make sure everything is labeled.

A great tool that I use in my personal beauty regiment is called a Facial-Flex. It is a face exerciser that I use every single day. It is used to help restore lost muscle tone and strengthen your chin, neck and cheek areas, making them noticeably tighter and smoother. It also promotes circulation for a healthy-looking glow. This is one of my best beauty suggestions and I hope you consider getting one. You can find this little gem by doing a search on the Internet.

Finally, I wanted to bring your full attention to yourself and your appearance. You must take notice of it and understand that you are still able to get dressed and look fantastic on a daily basis. Sure, you might have to make a few adjustments for your vision but the benefits will be immensely rewarding. When you look good you always feel better. Remember, hold your head up high. We are all God's creations, and we are beautiful! So, go on my friends, and Strut Your Stuff!

In Conclusion

Throughout these pages I have overwhelmingly stressed the importance of staying informed and educated about any type of resource or equipment that will help you live a fuller life. You must always maintain a deep-seated conviction of your own self-worth that will enable you to create a good plan of action to accomplish your goals. Do not wait for or depend on someone else to do this for you. You have to be bold, fearless, and determined. This mind-set will ultimately help you turn your dreams into reality. I know this can be scary, but "nothing ventured, nothing gained" is the truth.

For instance, if you are sure you need a special type of equipment, service, or whatever, fight for it! Things handed to people on a silver platter are a myth, or at least this is true in my own experience. If someone tells you no, go above or around them to accomplish your goals. You cannot passively sit on the sidelines and let the word "NO" crush your confidence or stop you from pursuing your dreams. Always remember that every challenge and nay-sayer we successfully face and defeat will help us conquer future obstacles in our path.

I also want to strongly reiterate that I believe miracles happen every single day. Look at all of the medical achievements and advancements that have occurred just in our lifetime. What is a normal procedure today was thought impossible in yesteryears. Your job is to tirelessly educate yourself on the latest medical research and brand-new techniques that are being developed for your specific vision problem. No one will be as diligent in this matter as you will be for yourself, because you are fighting for your own needs.

Let our life statement be "Never Give Up!" Using this as our motto, I know that we can all overcome the barriers and ignorance that is prevalent in our world. I want you to stay strong and never, ever falter in your belief and goal to have a better and productive life! The end result of anything will always lie in your heart and in your self-determination.

I am so very proud to be a part of such a great group of people that others label the visually impaired!

One final note: I would like to invite you to follow my web site www.nonieskorner.com, as well as my blog for any new updated information.

Resource Guide

General Resources:

National Federation of the Blind
Website: https://nfb.org
Telephone Number: 410-659-9314
NFB-News Line Staff: 1-866-504-7300

The American Foundation for the Blind
Website: www.afb.org
Phone: 212-502-7600

Division for the Blind and Physically Handicapped
Contact information varies by city and state.

The Department of Health and Human Services
Contact information varies by city and state.

Help Me! I Am Losing My Sight!

The Lions Club
Website: www.lionsclubs.org

The Red Cross
Website: www.redcross.org

Bureau of Engraving and Printing – free currency reader.
Website: www.bep.gov/uscurrencyreaderpgm

Product Vendors - Magnification

Ai Squared – makers of ZoomText.
Website: www.aisquared.com

Freedom Scientific – makers of MAGIC, JAWS and Open Book.
Website: www.freedomscientific.com

GW Micro – makers of Window Eyes.
Website: www.gwmicro.com

Dolphin – makers of Super Nova and screen reading software for cell phones.
Website: www.yourdolphin.com

Kurzweil Educational Systems – makers of Kurzweil 1000.
Website: www.kurzweiledu.com

Code Factory – maker of magnification and screen reading software programs for cell phones.
Website: http://codefactoryglobal.com

Nuance – maker of magnification and screen reading software programs for cell phones.
Website: www.nuance.com

esight – makers of electronic glasses which allow the visually-impaired to see.
Website: www.esighteyewear.com

Product Vendors – Readers

En-Vision America – makers of I.D. Mate, I.D. Mate Galaxy and ScripTalk.
Website: https://www.envisionamerica.com/

RNIB – makers of PenFriend – This product is available through a variety of websites.

Help Me! I Am Losing My Sight!

Franklin – makers of the Franklin Bill Reader.
Website: www.franklin.com

Orbit Research – makers of the Orbit iBill.
Website: www.orbitresearch.com

Millennium Compliance Corporation – makers of Talking RX
This product is available through a variety of websites.

Brytech – makers of Color Teller.
Website: www.brytech.com

Cobolt Systems – maker of Cobolt Color Detector.
Website: https://cobolt.co.uk

National Library Service
Website: www.loc.gov/nls/
Telephone Number: 1-800-424-8567
Direct Telephone Number: 202-707-5100

National Braille Press
Website: www.nbp.org
Telephone Number: 1-800-548-7323

American Council of the Blind – which provides the ACB Radio
Network.
Website: www.ACBRadio.org

Home Readers
Website: www.homereaders.com
Telephone Number: 1-877-814-7323

Media Access Group – providers of the Descriptive Video Service.
Website: http://main.wgbh.org

Product Vendors – Other

i-Robot Corporation (Roomba)
Website: http://store.irobot.com
Telephone Number: 1-800-727-9077

On-line Games

PCS Games
Website: www.pcsgames.net

Jim Kitchen Games
Website: http://www.kitchensinc.net/

GMA Games
Website: www.gmagames.com

DanZ Games
Website: www.danielzingaro.com

BSC Games
Website: http://blindcomputergames.com

Bavisoft
Website: www.bavisoft.com

All in Play
Website: http://allinplay.com

The AGRIP Project
Website: http://agrip.org.uk

Accessible Games
Website: www.accessiblegames.biz

Sports and Hobbies

Sports, Games and Recreation for the Blind and Physically Handicapped
Website: http://blindreaders.info/sports.html

American Blind Bowling Association
Contact: Judy Refosco at 724-745-5986
Address: 315 N. Main St., Houston, PA 15342

Blind Camps
Website: www.blindcamps.org

Space Camp
Website: www.spacecamp.com

United States Braille Chess Association
Website: www.americanblindchess.org

Handi Hams
Website: www.handiham.org

Volunteer Match
Website: www.volunteermatch.org

Blind Golf
Website: www.blindgolf.com

Music by Ear
Address: 704 Habersham Rd., Valdosta, GA 31602
Telephone Number: 229-249-0628

Help Me! I Am Losing My Sight!

PATH International
Website: www.pathintl.org

The Tandem Club of America
Website: http://tandemclub.org

Theater By The Blind
Website: www.tbtb.org

American Blind Skiing Foundation
Website: www.absf.org

Ski For Light
Website: www.sfl.org

Blind Sailing International
Website: www.blindsailinginternational.com

American Blind Skiers, Inc.
Address: 325 Wilshire Blvd., Santa Monica, CA 90403
Telephone Number: 213-828-5514

Handicapped Scuba Association
Website: www.hsascuba.com

National Beep Baseball Association
Website: www.nbba.org

SABAH
Website: www.sabahinc.org

Judo for Blind Athletes
Website: http://judoinfo.com

Goal Ball – Search for local opportunities.

Disabled Sports USA
Website: www.disabledsportsusa.org

Challenge Aspen
Website: http://challengeaspen.org

U.S. Adaptive Recreation Center
Website: http://usarc.org

United States Association of Blind Athletes
Website: www.usaba.org

British Blind Sport
Website: www.britishblindsport.org.uk

The International Blind Sports Federation
Website: www.ibsasport.org

Help Me! I Am Losing My Sight!

The Alliance for Disabled Sportsmen's Rights
Website: www.disabledrights.org
E-mail: Alliance@disabledrights.org

Books

"Getting Started With The iPhone. An Introduction for Blind Users" by Anna Dresner and Dean Martineau (National Braille Press) Available in print, Braille, and DAISY text.

About Darlene G. Smith

Having been visually-challenged for over forty years, Darlene knows firsthand how those diagnosed with a chronic eye disease may feel lost, alone, and even a little afraid. Committed to helping the vision impaired live happy, productive lives, she created Nonie's Korner LLC and its companion website www.nonieskorner.com.

With years of research and life experience, Darlene is committed to sharing her treasure trove of knowledge and creating how-to videos on her web site to benefit those who are dealing with poor vision.

She is a strong and determined woman who has not let eye disease define who she is and what she can accomplish. For example, in order to attend the University of Houston and receive her Bachelor of Science Degree, she hired several drivers over the course of three years to drive her 135 miles per day. She would not let blindness stand in her way of receiving that degree.

She wrote "Help Me I'm Losing My Sight" after so many friends and acquaintances showed a fervent interest in learning how she has mastered all the challenges associated with work, home and in all areas of life.

www.ingramcontent.com/pod-product-compliance
Lightning Source LLC
Chambersburg PA
CBHW080251030426
42334CB00023BA/2779